Sterile Processing, Invisible Culture "Reprocessed"

RICHARD CRAIG HUGHES

CONTENTS

ACKNOWLEDGMENTS

Thanks to all the people who took the time to teach me the science of Sterile Processing, and to everyone that helped me get through my first 30 years as a healthcare worker. I would also like to thank my wife Kelly for always supporting me and for helping me piece together the Sterile Prep Times issues for the 2nd Edition. Let's hope our efforts were not in vain.

1 THE INVISIBLE DEPARTMENT

Whatever possessed you to pick up this book or read it online? Well, the odds are overwhelming that you either work or have worked in a sterile processing department at some point in your life. Maybe you are curious about this new book on the market. Is it another instructional guide to add to your library of IAHCSSM or CBSPD manuals? What else could it be? Surely nobody would write a narrative about such a mundane subject as sterile processing. Well I have, and it's not nearly as mundane a subject as it was when I assembled my first minor instrument tray in 1990. Back then we assembled trays using instruments that would be described as "basic" in today's operating rooms. Instruments such as hemostats (criles), bone holders, needle holders, and the various types of retractors were our bread and butter. Today we deal with a wide array of instruments and medical devices that would make your head spin if you couldn't look up each and every one of them on a work station computer. Robotic arms and laparoscopic surgery have rendered the once-mighty curved crile all but obsolete. Think we had the luxury of computers back in 1990? Guess again. Our hospital was ahead of most, yet we didn't have a computerized instrument tracking system installed at each work station until the turn of the century. Everything was recorded using pen and paper products. Remember those? Of course fancy instruments and computers aren't the only improvements to sterile processing departments over the last three decades. Automatic washer-loading systems, automated endoscope reprocessors (AERs), multi-purpose ultrasonic/thermal/disinfector instrument washers, and so many other sophisticated devices and instruments. There is no doubt we are living in what my generation would consider the future.

Some things haven't changed about sterile processing departments, at least to my knowledge. They are still hidden so deeply inside the bowels of a hospital that the average person has no idea they exist or have ever existed. I can recount just about every hospital I've worked in, trained in, or interviewed for, and in each case I had to be personally escorted to Sterile Processing because there were no signs to point me there. And of course if you ask anyone else but a Central Service tech where the department is they merely shrug their shoulders and look at you like you have two heads. I've always thought that was more than a little strange. I mean we clean, assemble, package, sterilize, and re-distribute surgical instruments for the operating room. Every patient who goes under the knife is not only at the mercy of the surgeon but his or her team as well, and we are *vital* members of that team. Someone can always show you where the pharmacy is, the cafeteria, the x-ray department, ICU, and on a good day maybe even Endoscopy. But as for sterile processing, forget about it.

I experienced this phenomenon at my first sterile processing job in my hometown hospital. The department was not hard to find. In fact it was down the front hallway at the first corner, just past the cafeteria. The problem was there were no signs and nobody knew what "sterile prep" was, and that's what we were called in that facility. It was adjacent to the pharmacy. The sign by the doorway read "Pharmacy". There was also a sign nearby that pointed everyone to the cafeteria down the hall. The elevators were around the corner so there was another sign that read "Elevators" in big letters. But as for Sterile Processing...... forget about it. Guess you had to know somebody in the department in order to find it.

In the hospital where I most recently worked no one knew how to find our department except for the various instrument company reps who delivered and picked up their trays every other day and the folks in our sister department, Central Service. Even the administrators had to be reminded of whom and where we were when they did their semi-annual visitations of each department. It got pretty bizarre sometimes. Our hospital was a small cog in a large healthcare system so we received a lot of benefits without the burden of being so huge ourselves. For example there was a system-wide reporter who did weekly informational videos about interesting aspects of the hospital. He reported from a different campus each week. A few years ago he did a special report on our department. My manager was so stoked he personally escorted him throughout the various stages of our operation. I was working in decontam that day and I can tell you the reporter had no clue about what sterile processing techs do until that day. You know it's funny in a way. Everyone knows that surgeons use instruments to operate and everyone sees on television, through the news and various other shows that medical technology is expanding by leaps and bounds with each passing year. Yet very few people realize that all this expensive new instrumentation needs to be cleaned and reprocessed following each and every surgery. And because of that, even fewer can fathom that there is an entire department that focuses on the cleaning and sterilization of surgical instruments. We are in effect an *invisible department.*

I mentioned that our hospital was a small cog in a large system. The largest cog in the system was not far from us. It is the flagship hospital, a beautiful monster of a place on a gorgeous campus. A few years ago when our surgery department was undergoing some changes we were operating at roughly half our normal workload. The OR manager and Central Service manager together decided that rather than send people home as some companies do under such circumstances, they would send a few people each week to our flagship hospital. With blessings from the Sterile Processing manager in the larger facility, that is exactly what happened. As a result I got to experience working in one of the most state-of-the-art healthcare facilities in the country. I'll never forget the butterflies in my stomach while driving through one of their huge eight-story-plus parking garages looking for a space at 7:00 in the morning. It felt more like I was heading to a sporting event or a concert in downtown Orlando. After finding a space at the very top of the building I made my way through the various elevators, escalators, and hallways until finally arriving at the information desk. So far the entire experience reminded me of being on vacation in a multi-million dollar resort somewhere in the Caribbean. About the only amenities missing were the girls walking around in grass skirts. There was even a beautiful glass-covered walkway that passed over a parking lot and overlooked the spacious campus grounds below. It was hard to believe I was on my way to work. But headed to work I was, and when I asked the young lady at the information desk where the Sterile Processing department was everything began to return back to normal. She asked me to repeat which department I was looking for so I did. That's when I wish I had brought my GPS. It was down the hall, past a gigantic goldfish tank, turn right and go down another hallway past the courtyard, past the cafeteria and down another hallway, turn right and head down to……. the basement. That's right. The Sterile

Processing department in one of the largest, most majestic hospitals in the United States is in the basement. Good luck finding any signs; *invisible department.*

I once took a job as a sterile processing educator in another major facility in my home state of Florida, a trauma one hospital; drove all the way from our home in Vero to interview for the position. When I got to the information desk, instead of giving me directions to the department a young lady telephoned the Sterile Processing manager and told her I was there. The manager told the young lady she would meet me at the desk in ten minutes. As we walked toward the elevator that would lift us to the second floor my new manager, a middle aged woman with an obvious gift of gab, told me that she always met prospective employees at the information desk. She said it was easier than trying to tell them over the phone how to find the department. See the pattern here yet?

I could go on and on about hospitals with sterile

processing departments in remote corners, in basements, or hidden behind other departments, and those are just facilities where I have worked. Other techs have shared similar experiences about most of the hospitals they've worked in. Sterile Processing is an *invisible department.* It's a peculiar characteristic that might even defy explanation; or does it?

Could it be the reason we seem so invisible is because we never deal with the patient or their families in person? As I've previously stated, sterile processing is an integral element of surgery in any hospital. Together with Materials Management the Central Service department serves every single patient who walks or is wheeled through those doors. Yet we never actually get to meet them. When a patient or caregiver enters a hospital, he or she may become acquainted with healthcare workers from various other disciplines but the odds they will ever come in contact with a sterile processing tech are slim to none. That's our nature. We are an *invisible culture*; and that's fine. Our techs as a whole are not the most outgoing people in the workforce. I've even known a few co-workers through the years who actually preferred working in decontam over the other two alternatives (assembly and prep & pack). They enjoyed the seclusion and had a common belief that time seemed to pass by quicker because of the pace of the work. It takes a special kind of person to willingly gown up in hospital PPE and decontaminate bloody instruments for eight hours a stretch. We'll delve more into the type of people that fit the mold for this department in a later chapter. For now I would just say that if you are the kind of person who thrives on attention and/or careers that involve a lot of social contact, sterile processing might not be your forte'. Decontam especially would likely drive you mad.

The personal attributes of being independent and sometimes preferring to work alone are not exclusive to sterile processing techs of course. Other professions require those traits as well, such as auto mechanics, trucking, welding and fabrication, technical writing, and the list goes on. It's just this writer's opinion, but what sets sterile processing techs apart from the others is the *invisibility*. The auto mechanics, the truck drivers, the welders, et. al are out there every day plying their trades and serving the public in plain sight. Sterile processing techs on the other hand literally never see the light of day until their shift is over, and no one sees them except for their co-workers and the surgical techs who deliver the soiled instruments into decontam. And the kicker is no one else has even heard of them. My hope is that this book will be read by both sterile processing techs and the general public so that more people will become familiar with this burgeoning career. The complexity and technology in this field are growing by leaps and bounds and there is no way it can remain aloof. It is on the verge of breaking out and becoming one of the 21st century's biggest sleepers, ready for the rest of the world to discover. Ready to learn more about the department that supplies every single operating room in the free world with sterile instruments? A book about policies and procedures this is not. If that's what you are looking for you might better go online and Google IAHCSSM or AAMI, the governing bodies that together decide most of the policies in sterile processing departments across the country. This book is more of a 'Welcome to our world' kind of read. I set out to make it a book the lay person could use as a window to peer through the barriers that make this such an invisible culture. And I wanted the veteran technician to be able to relate and compare it to their own experiences and knowledge in the field. To that end, please accept my invitation into our world.

2 MAKING THE TRANSITION TO HOSPITAL WORK

Sterile processing is not the obscure career it used to be. More potential techs than ever before are learning about the assembly, packaging, and sterilization of surgical instrumentation shortly after high school graduation. They may be tipped off by a career counselor, friends who work in a hospital, or while job hunting on the internet. Prior to the recent surge in sterile processing technology, the majority of high school graduates assumed that the only non-degreed personnel in hospitals worked in the kitchen or environmental services. While it is true that the best hospital careers are still only available to college graduates, there are far more opportunities today than ever before for someone fresh out of high school or coming from another unrelated career.

What caused this sudden surge in sterile processing technology? You would have had to witness the changes in surgical technology in the past ten years or so to grasp the enormous changes. There have been leaps and bounds in virtually every facet of the job. Laparoscopic surgery, a relatively new alternative to the scalpel not long ago, fills up the daily surgery schedule in many hospitals today. Robotic surgery is heading in the same direction. The instrumentation used in these operations requires meticulous care throughout the entire cleaning and sterilization process. The use of ultrasonic cleaning sinks, computerized instrument washers, and sophisticated tracking systems call for competent employees to operate them. And that's where we come in.

How about you? Where did you come from? Did you start out flipping burgers or waiting tables? Perhaps you are pursuing a nursing degree and need to 'get your foot in the door' as they say. Maybe like the author you came from an outdoor career such as grounds maintenance or lawn care and were looking to work indoors for a change. Or maybe you just felt the calling as many health care workers do to help the sick. Whatever the reason you ended up working in a hospital, your first week there was most likely different from anywhere else you ever worked. I know mine was.

My hospital career began at the age of 31 in Vero Beach, Florida, "where the tropics begin." I concur. Not only do the tropics begin there but extreme summer heat abounds as well. After twelve years of working in the great outdoors manicuring golf courses and customers' lawns, and with my dermatologist's blessings, I decided to look for another career, preferably indoors. For some reason the idea of shooting x-rays kept popping up in my mind so I began researching how one might go about finding a job in a hospital. Funny how God works but it turned out that my sister had just landed a job at our local hospital only a couple of months before my search began, in the Human Resources department no less! She started the ball rolling in my favor and the next thing you know I was interviewing for a job in Sterile Prep (whatever that is!). During my first few years in the hospital I learned *a lot*. Let me share just a few of the things I learned in those first five years, at least the ones I can remember. After all, we are talking about almost thirty years ago as of this writing.

I learned that *saying* you want to be something and actually *becoming* the person you want to be are two different things entirely.

I learned that one should research a career to the point of exhaustion before diving into it without knowing much about it. Finding out that one is not compatible with a potential career early can save a lot of disappointment down the road.

I learned about *patience*, or should I say *Patience* with a capital *P*. As in sometimes it takes **years** to accomplish what you thought would take months. And it's not always about accomplishments. Patience with people can be just as challenging. Not everyone is going to jump on the bandwagon and help you accomplish your goals unless there is something tangible in it for them too. Expecting everyone and everything in life to fall into place according to your plans is not only naïve but selfish as well. When one realizes that just isn't going to happen, it's all a part of that elusive and ambiguous process we call maturity.

There are plenty of ways to make a living when you are young and ambitious but it is up to the individual as to which way is best. Jobs that require hard labor for meager wages are more abundant than jobs that offer opportunities for advancement and personal growth along with an attractive salary. Yet an honest day's work rewarded by decent but modest pay will always be one of the best character builders in our society. Another thing I learned on my own, and it is best if you learn this one on your own, is to *never give up*. Throughout our careers we always hear this cliché, whether it comes from a coach, a big brother, a father, or anyone else who has an impact on our lives, and it is one of the best codes to live by. But we have to learn it on our own and it has to come by trial and error. There may be a few gifted and special people who have succeeded in life with very few trials and errors. We have all known at least a few people who seemed to have everything going for them and could do no wrong. They always made the right choices and we never knew how they did it. Well they could have been hiding their true story or they may have been extremely blessed, but the rest of us have to learn by trial and error. Never give up.

In the hospital there are (generally speaking) two types of work, and to put it bluntly one is a job and the other is a career. One is available to anyone seeking to get their foot in the door of a hospital after graduating from high school or working at a job unrelated to healthcare. The other is available only to college graduates with a degree in business or allied health.

These are the two main types of jobs available at any hospital.

Whether you have been training for a career in the medical field or are coming in fresh from an entirely different walk of life, working in a hospital is going to challenge you in ways that you may have never considered. For instance if you thought there were too many rules and regulations at your last job you will be amazed by their sheer numbers in a hospital. There is so much to learn during the first year of employment no matter which healthcare career you have chosen, and that doesn't even include all the new information you will have to learn in your chosen field. As you might guess hospitals have to conform to the strictest of health codes in order to keep their license and not have to pay hefty fines. Two of the most notorious health care advocates in the United States, the Agency for Health Care Administration (AHCA) and The Joint Commission, conduct rigid inspections each year to make sure every nationally accredited facility is safe for patients. If you are curious as to just how stringent the regulations are at a typical American hospital just check out their respective websites: www.ahcancal.org and www.jointcommission.org.

All of this is not to downplay all the regulations that abound on other jobsites such as restaurants, road construction, the hotel business, NASA, the airlines, manufacturing, etc. Each of these has their own watchdog agencies they must satisfy as well. The point is if you work in a hospital you *will* be held accountable for being familiar with the expectations of both AHCA and The Joint Commission. It's not a secondary requirement as it is in many other careers; rather it takes precedence over your actual job duties. They are serious about this. MSDS sheets, HIPAA legislation, safety codes, fire safety, and Policies and Procedures are all required reading for the new hires in a hospital. Although it's true that no one could ever recite all this info off the top of their head, they had better know where to find it when asked by an official AHCA inspector.

If you are accustomed to working outdoors you are among a group that will notice perhaps the greatest disparity between your former job and a career in the hospital. There are so many different types of outdoor careers it would be all but impossible to name the top priority of business of each and every one of them. For example, the most important duty of a firefighter is to save lives; same goes for a paramedic and a police officer. The most important duty of a construction worker is to do quality work so that the finished product is as good as it can possibly be. Now watch this. The most important duty of a hospital worker is to *stay clean*. I'm not making this up. One of the slogans of one of the hospitals I worked for was always *"Wash your hands!"* And they stressed this because of the importance of keeping one's hands clean in the closed hospital environment. *"Primum non nocere"* is a Latin phrase that means *"first, do no harm."* It is part of the Hippocratic Oath that doctors must take while they are still in medical school, and it basically means that the most important duty of a physician is to not harm the patient. The potential for harming patients in any hospital is most common through the transmission of diseases and germs by way of cross-contamination and human contact. And so the theory goes that the best method for eliminating the spread of germs and disease through human contact is to wash your hands, and this method is used beyond anything you could imagine coming from the outside world. As hospital workers we wash our hands *before* doing a job and *after* completing that job; *before* touching a patient and *after* touching that patient; *before* shaking someone's hand and *after* shaking someone's hand; *before* using the restroom and *after* using the restroom; *before* entering our own department and *after* leaving our department. Get the picture? The idea is to stop the spread of germs and diseases inside the hospital and to avoid any HAIs (healthcare-acquired infections), formerly known as nosocomial infections. There are various other methods used in the hospital to avoid the spread of infections. You will learn those in time but keeping your hands clean is THE most important one.

Another anomaly you may notice in your transfer from outdoor work to the hospital setting is the way your fellow workers are treated. Depending upon what career you just left your co-workers may have dug ditches, mowed yards, trimmed hedges, sprayed pesticides on lake banks, or a host of other jobs that wear a person out in the drenching heat of summer. They were probably treated by their bosses according to how hard they worked and how well they did their jobs on a daily basis. In many jobs speed is a factor in how workers are rated by both their superiors and co-workers as well. In other words **respect** is earned through a lot of hard work and goes hand in hand with quality and efficiency. Nobody gets off easy lest they risk the danger of being ridiculed by their cohorts for being a 'brown-noser.'

A career in healthcare is a little different. For instance a new hire who is caring, sincere, kind, and gentle may be valued more than someone on staff who gets the job done but doesn't act very thoughtful to others. In the healthcare field a little kindness goes a long way. Perhaps management sees a potential caregiver in every new hire; maybe they don't want to take any chances with workers who might anger the patients or their families. Whatever the reason, your new co-workers are going to have different work habits than your buddies on the old work crew, and some of them might flat out irk you. Case in point:

Some time ago I worked a couple of years at a truck stop after responding to an ad on TV. They were looking for diesel mechanics, no experience needed. They would provide the training. My dad had been an auto mechanic in his younger days and I had always wanted to follow in his footsteps, but he never encouraged me in that direction. It wasn't the type of career he had wanted for either of his sons. Working on cars was hard, filthy, and sometimes dangerous work. Yet even in middle age I still yearned to fill his shoes. With his blessings I applied and got the job. Well I found out early on that an apprentice mechanic has to change a lot of tires and do a ton of lube jobs before he gets to be an official diesel mechanic. And that's mostly what I did for the whole two years I was there. I did have the opportunity to change out some batteries and alternators, do some welding, and even installed new thermostats in a huge Caterpillar engine once, but my bread and butter was what they called the 'PM Special.' There was something like 120 points on each big rig I was supposed to check and/or lubricate, and check each one off as I did it. Brakes, windshield wipers, checking the tires for air, cooling system, batteries, etc.; each system had to be checked and checked off. The first PM I performed on a tractor-trailer took about three hours. When I brought the finished checklist to the head mechanic he just shook his head in disgust, barely even looking up at me.

"You're going to have to get a lot faster than that!" is all he said; not 'good job' or 'great effort' or even 'not bad for your first truck.' Nope, it was "You're going to have to get a lot faster than that."

So I did. I got a *lot* faster, and better too, with time.

By the end of my rookie year I had whittled the time of a PM Special down to about an hour. The head mechanic was happy, the boss was happy, and the truckers started asking for me whenever they pulled into the shop for a lube job and inspection. I was thorough, fast, and I cared about my work. And that's what it took to please those truckers. And in case you didn't know, truckers don't let just *anyone* work on their big rigs.

Compare that with sterile processing, a job I have been doing now for about thirty years. I've probably cleaned at least 90% of the different types of instrumentation ever crafted since the dawn of the 21st century. Robotics, orthopedic trials, laparoscopic forceps, fiber-optics, everything from flexible scopes to flexible reamers; you name it and I've probably cleaned and sterilized it. And yet for all of that experience, my supervisors would still prefer that I spend 45 minutes cleaning a set of robotic arms, of which there are usually only seven or eight, than to shorten that time to around 20 minutes, even if I guarantee that they will be clean.

And that is only a pre-cleaning prior to putting them into an ultrasonic washer that flushes out the lumens *again*, rinses, and then thermally disinfects them in a 45-minute cycle. I mean I know these instruments will be used on patients. Believe me I *get* that. But it's just so hard sometimes to perform overkill on a cleaning job and spend twice as much time as necessary when there comes a point in the cleaning phase when *clean is clean*. They are surgical instruments, yes. But in a way it is still like washing your car or your motorcycle or even your bicycle. If you've gone over the whole thing twice diligently, being ever so careful as to not miss the slightest nook or cranny, is it going to get any cleaner if you go over it a third time? Okay, end of rant. It's not going to change the IFU's of any instrumentation and it's certainly not going to change the way your supervisor feels about how you need to clean everything. Just thought you should know what you will be facing if you are considering a career in sterile processing.

But back to my original point here: There are those

who won't even be fazed by the meticulous cleaning requirements in decontam or in any other area of the hospital because they have never worked in a job where competing for time was the norm. Those are the people who are going to drive you crazy as they labor over a tiny simple device for what seems like way too long as you shake your head and think 'I could clean that in about thirty seconds.' But it doesn't end there. Mark my words, they will get praise and kudos all day long for their slothful ways while all you get is criticism and scorn for what you have always thought was called efficiency. I feel you my friend. It's not going to be easy for you to make the adjustment. Just buck up and remember that your other job was probably just a job. This one can be made into a career. Remember that and you just might make it in the hospital business.

So there you have it, some tips for those who are making the transition into hospital work for the first time. As a bonus to you future sterile processing technicians, here are a few guidelines for your job interview to help you ask the right questions. There are a few things you need to know about the job you are applying for and the person(s) who will have the power to either make or break you in your new job. If you really want to learn the trade, not one of these is a game changer but knowing what you are getting into can sometimes make the transition go a bit smoother. So here we go. Questions you might want to ask at a sterile processing job interview:

1) What is the bosses-to-workers ratio? Why is this important? You're pretty smart; you should be able to figure this one out. If you came from an outdoor job where there was one boss on the job sight and eight or more workers, you might be in for a real shocker when you get your first sterile processing job. It is not uncommon for the bosses to outnumber the regular workers in this department. Think I'm making this up? One of the Sterile departments where I worked was

going through a management transition and had no less than five bosses on hand while there were only three of us doing the actual work. I kid you not. Do you have any idea what that would be like? About the only way to describe it is this: pretend you are driving to another state in the company mini-van with five passengers, each of whom is either a department supervisor or manager, and therefore has the authority to tell you to go wherever they want you to go. Pretty uncomfortable, wouldn't you think? Just out of curiosity ask the interviewer the bosses-to-workers ratio.

2) Ask about any special rules or policies you should know about that might become aggravating after awhile, such as mandatory masks for facial hair, mandatory flu shots, working overtime, and anything else you can think of that might bother you enough to consider finding another place of employment.

3) Check the job description thoroughly and if there are any questions about a particular assignment, make sure you understand what is expected of you. Some sterile processing departments have to clean a lot more equipment than others. Items such as I.V. infusion pumps, code carts and code drawers, and even cots from the Emergency Department are fair game in some Sterile Processing departments. Find out ahead of time so there are no big surprises should you land the job.

Those are just a sample of the questions you should ask at your job interview. Of course you will also be interested in their benefits, holiday pay policy, sick time, and merit and cost of living raises. Good luck with your interview and your big transition into hospital work. I hope it is everything you had expected it to be, and if it's not, well hopefully you didn't burn any bridges in your last line of work. But give it a chance. Hang in there and you just might find hospital work to be one of the most rewarding and fulfilling experiences in your lifelong career.

3 WHAT ARE YOU DOING HERE?

It's fair to say that a good percentage of workers stay in their careers long after they begin to feel out of place. A word of caution here: You really shouldn't stick around long in a sterile processing department once that feeling overtakes you. It's not fair to the patient, nor is it fair to your co-workers, and quite frankly it's not fair to you either. The tasks of decontamination, assembly, and sterilization of surgical instruments are crucial and require diligence, focus, and patience. But above all they demand a positive attitude. Negativity in such a small social circle as the sterile processing department spreads like a virus. Tech burnout is common in this career after a few years on the job. Tasks become routine and repetitive, and the need for some time away from the hospital environment is real. A long weekend every now and then or perhaps even a week or two off once or twice a year, if your manager permits it, should suffice to refresh your spirits. But if you return from vacation and still feel that depressing feeling of being trapped in your job, well that is called burnout, and it may be time to start looking for another way to make a living.

But what if you decide to stay? What is it about this job, this career if you will, that makes some people keep coming back for more? Is there a certain type of personality trait or traits that embrace the sterile processing environment? Is this now a viable career that one can actually plan a life around, such as working in the hospital pharmacy or lab? Let's take a closer look and maybe we can find the answers to these questions and learn about what kind of person makes the ideal sterile processing technician.

In the first chapter and randomly throughout this book, I have mentioned in one context or another that by the time this manuscript is published I will have worked thirty years in central service, twenty-five of which were spent in sterile processing. Now I don't know if that qualifies as a long time in the grand scheme of things but it is exactly half my life as I write this. In fact the only other careers I have toiled at for even close to that extent are golf course maintenance and lawn care. By the age of 40 I thought I'd be mowing grass for the rest of my life. For a more detailed look at the mowing life you can check out my book *"Mowing at the Master's Level"* (2018), available on **Amazon.com**. Luckily I'd been working as a sterile processing tech on the evening shift at our local hospital since the age of 30 so I had an out and took it. For close to ten years I carried out lawn care or golf course maintenance duties five days a week until 3:00 each afternoon, then headed to the hospital and changed into scrubs to finish out the day as a sterile processing tech. The two jobs could not have been more diverse; eight hours of sweating it out in the hot Florida sun followed by a full shift of working with surgical instrumentation. Perhaps that was the only reason I was able to work the two back to back jobs for such a long time; their diversity. In a strange way they might have complemented each other by virtue of their extreme polarity. They certainly didn't have too much in common. One job required strength, stamina, and love of the Florida outdoors. The other demanded dedication to detail, staying clean, and a tolerance for working inside of windowless rooms with no chance of seeing daylight for hours at a time. And that brings us back to the first question. What is it about sterile processing that makes some people want to stick with it for a few years, a decade or so, or even a lifetime? I suppose the short answer would be that there is a niche for everyone in the workforce, but let's take a closer look at some of the virtues of a sterile processing career.

First of all it must be said that although the job is routine it is actually a composite of three distinct operations rolled into one: decontamination, assembly, and sterilization. If your hospital rotates the different tasks throughout the week, as most do, you should never have to repeat any one of them more than once, assuming you are properly staffed. This characteristic makes it a much more attractive entry level hospital job than say environmental services, nutritional services (i.e. cafeteria), or central supply. By "properly staffed" I mean that no one should have to work in decontam more than two days a week unless of course we are talking about a really small department. I've worked in departments so small they had only one full-time tech on staff and the surgical techs had to help clean their own dirty instruments when the OR got really busy. If working alone is your cup of tea you might want to look into finding a job at a really small facility. For the rest of us a hospital with anywhere between 200 and 300 beds is average for a small community; 500 to 600 beds for a larger city, and on up to the mega-size facilities that grace the landscapes of cities like Pittsburgh, Chicago, Miami, and Boston. Large or small there is an indescribable feeling of purpose that takes over your spirit from day one as a sterile processing tech; even more so if you are a transplant from a totally different walk of life, such as landscaping or building maintenance. It's not that those other jobs are less meaningful or unnecessary. On the contrary, the older I get the more I realize that every job that someone is willing to pay for is necessary and meaningful to somebody, and therefore deserves the respect of its workers. It's just that once your new boss or manager explains to you exactly what your purpose is as a sterile processing tech, your first reaction is generally something like 'You mean trays that I assemble are going to be used in *surgery; by doctors?*' It is difficult to fathom at first that surgeons with 8-plus years of med school will use instruments prepared by you, who only a week or so ago were mowing grass or planting trees for a living. I think the person who holds on to that initial feeling of disbelief that something he or she created will be used to heal patients on an operating table, will last the longest in this profession.

The idea that sterile processing is a noble profession is not too far-fetched. After all, as many in the business would be quick to remind the layperson, surgeons could not operate without sterile instruments. Having said that, there are sterile processing techs who have been doing this job for ten years, perhaps twenty, and have yet to step foot inside an operating room or even a patient's room for that matter. Indeed there are some SP departments that do not require or permit their techs to leave the immediate surroundings for any reason while on the clock. Some people are okay with this; others get claustrophobic. Regardless departmental policy must be adhered to. If this sounds like an important detail, you might want to ask about things like this during the job interview. The fact of the matter is, whether this job is hailed as a noble one or not, there is generally very little if any patient contact in this career. What makes it noble is that a responsible sterile processing technician has to put himself or herself into the patients' and doctors' shoes (or socks as it were) every single moment of every day while on duty. That is the only way to do this job right. So there is the nobility aspect that appeals to those who otherwise might be working in retail or performing home services such as laying carpet or floor tile, or hanging light fixtures. In other words, sterile processing turns the average blue collar worker into a scrub-wearing physician's assistant of sorts.

Aside from that it's just a job that has its virtues and pitfalls. You're indoors every day, which is a plus if you don't like dealing with extreme weather conditions, a minus if you love being outdoors. The whole department is air conditioned and pretty comfortable. In fact one has to really be pushing it to work up a sweat in the assembly area or prep and pack. And then there is decontam. Ah yes, decontam. The very word strikes terror into some who have built up an absolute phobia or hatred for the nastiest job of this three-phase career. It's noisy. It's hot and stuffy with all the PPE one has to wear while cleaning and sorting soiled instruments. And the work is non-stop throughout the day no matter how many cases were on the board first thing in the morning. Not to mention that if you do happen to prick yourself or unwittingly slice a finger with a sharp instrument, count on spending the better part of the rest of your day in the Emergency Room filing an incident report and preventing the spread of infection. It's not that everyone agrees across the board that decontam is the worst job in sterile processing. There will always be those who would rather be back there than out front on the clean side. It's just like any other occupation in that some workers want to do the nasty chores for whatever reason. As I have done in other books, I will once again use my old friend and former golf course maintenance co-worker as an example here. At 47 years old, Jack was one of the older gentlemen on an otherwise youthful crew of about seven guys. Double that number if you include both the North and South courses. Because of his age and seniority on the golf course he could have easily been the designated fairway unit operator, or tee mower, tractor driver or any other job where he could have spent the majority of the work week sitting on a machine. Instead most of the younger guys held those positions. Jack had put in a request early on in his career to do most of the weedeating, lake bank mowing, and trash pickup on the course. It seems that when he lived up north he had some type of office job. I never asked about the details but it must have been somewhat of a high-stress position because his doctor told him if he didn't quit his job he would be heading for a heart attack. Stressed out and overweight, he brought his wife and two young kids down to Florida in the early 1970's and decided to work his extra weight off as a golf course maintenance crew worker. It must have worked because Jack retired from the golf course at the youthful age of seventy after almost thirty years of hand mowing greens, weedeating, and fly-mowing lake banks. My point is that everyone has their reasons for wanting to do the dirty work. I've worked in decontam as much as anyone with twenty-five years of experience in the field and can attest to at least a couple of niceties about the job worth mentioning. For one, like mowing lake banks and weedeating in the deep roughs of a golf course, nobody bothers you in decontam. Heck nobody wants to go back there during the course of a busy day. It's usually jam-packed full of dirty instruments and case carts. So if you don't like being bothered decontam is a great place to spend a day. Another nice feature is that in most facilities you get to have a radio back there playing your favorite music, so especially if you are by yourself in a smaller hospital, you can pretend you're working in your own workshop at home. Just imagine you're not wearing all the suffocating PPE.

There are a few good reasons people decide to stay in this career. But instead of going into detail about every little benefit of working in sterile processing let's take a look at what kind of person is most likely to stay. We've already established there is no patient contact and practically no contact with anyone else in the hospital outside of your own department. That narrows it down to people who don't mind working day in and day out with the same close-knit clan, similar to working in a machine shop or other type of plant where you may not see the light of day until your shift is over. It would help if you like working with your hands too. It's not necessary to be creative, as a sterile processing tech does not actually build or *create* anything per se. Wrapping instrument trays does however require a certain amount of finesse. Some never pick it up. They might work in this career for ten years and their trays still look more like a five-year-old's failed attempt at wrapping large Christmas presents. So in that respect you might say it does require a certain amount of talent to pack instrument trays. Same goes with the assembly process. Someone with very little finger dexterity who is all thumbs is going to deliver some pretty ugly trays to the OR. Still the bottom line is they are clean and sterile at the end of the process. I'm sure the surgical techs appreciate trays that are nice and neat with everything in its place but there is no need to turn it into an art show. As far as decontam goes the key word back there these days is *meticulous*. Back when I first started working in a hospital in 1990 the decontam process was more akin to being a dishwasher in a busy restaurant than anything else. That's a pretty accurate analogy and I know that from experience, having worked in three restaurant kitchens prior to finding a career in sterile processing. Nowadays you can throw that comparison away. With the advent and widespread usage of laparoscopic instruments, cannulated screw sets, robotic arms, flexible scopes, and a host of other new classifications of instruments, working in a modern day decontam is more like working in a clean room in a semiconductor manufacturing plant. And this is one of the problems facing sterile processing managers and recruiters today. How do they hire and then hold on to techs whose job is to know every detail about complex surgical instruments, when their budget only allows them to pay wages slightly more than that of a high school janitor? No doubt there are a lot of unhappy sterile processing techs who blame their managers or hospitals for the low wages they receive. The fact is the machinery required to clean and sterilize all the complex gadgetry used in surgery today is so expensive that only the most elite hospitals can afford to pay for it and still have enough left over in the budget to pay good wages to enough staff. And that is probably the biggest single problem facing most sterile processing departments of the present era. The solution is not for me to say as I'm neither a manager nor a consultant and don't get paid big bucks for solving problems of that magnitude. But it is clearly a tradeoff. Aside from the most prestigious hospitals and hospital systems in the world, all the rest have to choose where their money will best be spent. Do they invest in high dollar high-tech machinery or pay their employees decent wages for their uncommon skill sets? It's not an easy decision. The specialized equipment used for cleaning instruments, case carts, and utensils these days makes the job much easier to bear than manual cleaning. But a decontam full of fancy washers will not clean much without competent staff to operate them. And like a new car they won't stay new for long. They get used and abused and need maintenance and repairs. The older they get the more repairs they need. So it's a tough decision, one I'm sure only the most savvy department heads are qualified to make.

And that leads us to what might be the most important quality of a sterile processing tech: *dedication*. It might sound trite but without dedication a new tech may find it difficult to find a reason to stay in this job when the going gets tough. No it's not the toughest job on the market, not even close. But without a sense of direction or purpose this job can sometimes feel meaningless and senseless. Case in point: You come into work one day to find out that not only is one of your key co-workers out sick, but another is on vacation and your supervisor is stuck in traffic and will be late. There was only one person on the night shift, and he or she walked into a big mess and couldn't get much done on his/ her own. So the mess is passed on to you and one of your remaining co-workers, and it looks like surgery is going to be busy again today. This is not an uncommon scenario. In fact it's practically a normal day. It takes all day to get caught up with yesterday's workload and meanwhile today's is steadily pouring through the washers with only half of the staff needed to get the job done properly. Welcome to sterile processing. I know it probably shouldn't be this way but like I said before, because of the high cost of instrumentation and machinery there is not much left to go around and that's just basic economics. So if you don't have a purpose or a cause that you can dedicate yourself and your work to, it may be difficult to make it through days like this. At the very least you need a good team of co-workers to help you get through the tough times and help you answer questions like "What am I doing here?"

4 WORKING TOGETHER IN THE STERILE ENVIRONMENT

A sterile processing department is similar to just about every other nursing unit in the hospital in more ways than one. First and foremost, every nursing unit in every hospital has one top priority and they drill this into your head almost every day of your life as a nurse: to serve the patient. The better hospitals teach their sterile processing techs the same thing. In practice this means that whenever one is cleaning an intricate, time consuming instrument and is urged to rush through the process without careful inspection, one must always remember this instrument is not being used to turn screws in a house or a car. It will be introduced into a patient's body; their vital organs and extremities; blood and tissue; heart and lungs. When you can imagine each instrument you touch and visually inspect being inserted into a patient's wide open surgical wound at a time when they are completely at the mercy of the surgeon, his skills, and his instruments, then and only then can you be trusted as a sterile processing tech. This is why we in the field secretly know that our compensation may not be anywhere near that of an RN but our job is equally important. Without clean and sterile instruments the patient's health would go downhill immediately following surgery. So we share that level of involvement in patient care with the nursing department.

There is another characteristic that sterile processing techs share with nurses almost universally, across the board. The majority of them are female. And anyone that has ever been in a hospital as a patient or visitor has probably noticed that an overwhelming majority of nurses are female as well, which begs the question: Do females make the best caregivers? Everyone reading this is already nodding their heads in agreement, a hands-down "Oh yeah." I didn't bring up the idea to make a point or start an argument. I simply wanted to state a fact and give a fair picture of the demographics of our "trade" if you will, so that if you are thinking about a career in sterile processing, especially if you're a guy, you're getting a little heads up as to what you might expect in the way of co-workers.

There are of course countless scenarios when it comes down to the demographics of any given sterile processing department. Whenever you have a career where gender is not a factor in the selection of employees, there is no telling what kind of "blend" you might get. Sociologists would have a field day studying the various nuances of employee behaviors, especially in a large department. A successful healthcare team depends upon the cooperation and communication between its members. Nowhere is this as evident as in a surgical services department, and that includes sterile processing.

As I have indicated in other chapters and in other books as well, the bulk of my work experience other than that of a central service tech for 30 years was in lawn and golf course maintenance. During those 15 years or so there was very little contact with workers of the opposite gender. In fact one of my older co-workers on the golf course once commented that working there was the closest thing he had encountered to being in the service since he got out of the army, and he was likely either a World War II or Korean War veteran. I'm not sure if he was in the armored division or something similar where they drove heavy equipment every day, but he did say it reminded him of the camaraderie that existed between soldiers in the same company. That was the same camaraderie we shared with the other workers on the golf course and it was also the same on the lawn maintenance crews. There was a real sense of watching out for your buddies, of having each other's backs. When I started working at my first hospital that sense of being surrounded every day by my buddies was gone. That's why I am mentioning this and giving a heads up to those who come to the hospital from working outdoors. I know from experience you are going to go through some major changes in the way you respond to your new job. It is both psychologically and physically different from what you are used to and there will be many adjustments that have to be made.

A significant difference is the one I have already mentioned; that of transitioning from a primarily all-male work crew to a mixture that can sometimes be closer to all-female. This changes the atmosphere in the workplace in ways that sometimes rival the big change from outdoors to indoors. Now here is where it gets tricky. I'm going to try to explain some of the ways that working with women is unlike working with men. Mind you this is coming from a male author who has a Bachelor's degree in Psychology from the University of Central Florida. And that is not to say I know *a lot* about psychology; on the contrary holding a Bachelor's in Psychology means that I only know that I know *very little* about psychology, *especially* about women. But I have undoubtedly learned more about women in my twenty-five years of working in sterile processing than I could ever learn in college, even if I had graduated with a PhD.

If this chapter were a thesis for a Master's degree in Social Psychology I would have probably given it the same title. The big difference is I would have had to do a lot of research on the subject, cite a ton of articles, and use a bunch of footnotes, and that is not what this book is all about. As you know, it's a collection of information the author has deemed useful to anyone interested in the field of sterile processing. I have tried my best to make this an unbiased account of the subject but having said that, it is bound to come off as a personal account of a worker who has struggled in the same career for thirty years. So be it; it is what it is. So enough of the long intro, let us dive into this intriguing topic. How can we all work together, male and female, the young and the not-so-young, and every race and religion on God's green Earth, to make our sterile processing departments a success for the patients and employees alike? There are no simple answers but this is the issue facing a growing number of hospitals as America's workforce grows more diverse with each passing year. Yet for many sterile processing departments the answer is in the question. The secret to getting along is to focus on the patients.

The best reason I can think of to focus on the patients is that not everyone that works in a hospital is a Christian. If they were, the obvious choice would be to love one another as Jesus did and as He asked us to do. For those who do not follow Christ's example it is suggested they work each day as if one of their family members were being operated on and they are cleaning and sterilizing the instruments for surgery. In this way it is thought a tech can concentrate on doing a proper job regardless of any distractions, even if those distractions come from his or her co-workers. Okay, what am I talking about here? Why and how would your co-workers be causing distractions while everyone is supposed to be working on delivering a quality product to the OR each day? I saw it best summed up in a short but excellent article written by Dr. Barton Goldsmith, PhD in the online magazine *Psychology Today* (Aug. 31, 2010). The article was titled "Men, Women, Emotion and Communications" and the good doctor said,

"It is interesting to note that women think and feel at the same time, while men can only think or feel. And based on most men's reluctance to embrace their feminine side, it's no wonder they do their level best to stay in their heads."

Wow. That's what a PhD can do for you folks. He just explained more in those two sentences than I could have done in two pages; saved me a lot of typing. I could almost end the chapter right here and leave every reader, both men and women alike, nodding their heads and saying "He got that right!" But I guess I should continue on and try to explain how that short synopsis pertains to everyday work in an average sterile processing department. Okay, here's the thing, and let me point out that I am generalizing here. I am open minded enough to know that there is not one thing anyone can say about gender differences that holds true 100% in every case. Yet it has been my observation throughout the years that women find it *much* easier to work an eight-hour shift if they are able to talk freely to their co-workers. Not trying to be flippant about it or anything, it's just something I've learned to take for granted whenever I go to a new job or different hospital. It used to bother me but now I just chalk it up as a feminine characteristic and not something that women do to purposely anger the men in the department. Nor do they talk excessively in order to slow down the work progress. In most cases they simply perform better when they are allowed to talk to their co-workers as much as possible. There are exceptions of course. Just as there are men with feminine traits, including the need or desire to talk while they work, there are also women who prefer silence over conversation, especially when the job requires concentration. And then there are those tasks in sterile processing that require total concentration by every tech across the board, both male and female. One of the last hospitals I worked at utilized a computer tracking system that was pretty simple to operate in the assembly and decontam phases. All that was required was to scan each instrument tray into the system as it passed through each phase. Sterilization was a different story. It took total concentration to keep track of the load numbers, biological readouts, sterilization exposure times and methods, and equipment failures. Virtually every one of us, when assigned to sterilization for the day, would forego almost all conversation, especially while we were putting information into the computer. So you see it is possible.

Aside from the talking thing, I have found that both men and women are pretty much on equal ground in this profession. Decontam is physically demanding for both genders, young and old alike. The required PPE along with the volume and type of work involved make for a rather stressful environment. Like I have said before, there are much tougher jobs on the market but decontam is usually the toughest one in any sterile processing department. As for wrapping instrument trays, women usually have a knack for wrapping things but it's not a skill that men cannot pick up with practice as well. Assembly is also a skill that anyone can learn. Men and women who come from a background of working with tools will naturally find it easier to work with the various laparoscopic instruments that need to be taken apart in decontam and re-assembled on the clean side. The true beauty of this career is how anyone can learn to excel in it no matter what their background, gender, or skill set. It's not as simple as it used to be but it is still quite teachable and learnable.

The smooth running of any department does not depend solely on the knowledge and skills of its workers, however important that may be. As we all know it depends more on how everyone works **together**. If men truly want to get along with women in the workplace they must learn to speak their "language." When a man finds himself outnumbered by women on any given day in sterile processing, say for example in the assembly area, he soon finds out the topics females like to talk about: family, their kids, grandkids if applicable, relationships, clothes, shopping, and perfumes are just a few of their favorite subjects. I think we all know what most men like to talk about, but just so we are all on the same page: sports, their kids, grandkids, different jobs they used to have, and past experiences with their buddies. Some guys still like talking about cars but not nearly as much as we did in the old days when muscle cars were the main subject. The trick to conversation between the two genders at work is to find common ground. Current affairs are always on people's minds every day but there is so much bad news in the world today that it can get depressing just like the news, so some co-workers may just try to change the subject to something more lighthearted. Everyone likes to talk about their kids and what they've been up to lately. Here's a good one: if you want to strike up a conversation with a woman just ask her how she is feeling; women love to relate their feelings. They are all about feelings and emotions. Want to break the silence with one of the guys in the department? Try asking about his favorite hobby if you know what it is. If not, ask him what he likes to do in his spare time. Men love spare time. It's something we cherish. There's never enough of it. While we are on the subject of men and women trying to speak in each other's language, have you ever noticed the difference in how a single woman tries to initiate conversation with a single man and vice-versa? Women tend to be more *suttle* in their approach if you will, when asking personal questions. For example, when a single man wants to find out if a new female co-worker is single or married he might come right out and ask her,

"So.....are you married?"

Conversely, a woman would **never** ask a man that question. Any woman who asks the new guy if he is married or single must be flirting with him, and that is exactly how he is going to interpret it. So a woman has to look for all the "signs" and she usually does this before approaching him for the first time. The most obvious one is a wedding ring. But some sterile processing departments are so strict these days they don't even allow employees to wear rings. If there are no obvious signs she might approach him with a couple of casual questions to test the waters, such as:

"Does your wife (or girlfriend) work at a hospital too?" or

"You sure do have a great sense of humor. Your wife must really appreciate that."

By the way, women really do appreciate a man with a good sense of humor. It's important in the home and equally so on the job in order to break up the monotony of a routine day. Men who are quick witted and humble will make a lot of friends in this career. If you have ever worked in sterile processing you know what I mean. Equipment breakdowns, work overload, and being understaffed are common in this line of work, and every department can use a man who rolls with the punches. Women also appreciate a man who can help carry the extra workload without complaining when the department is understaffed. Most women will freely admit they enjoy having a few good men around, especially when there is a lot of work to do. Some may even prefer more men than women in the department. But many in this field enjoy working with other women; that is one of their favorite things about the job.

And what about some qualities that men appreciate in the women they work with? Believe it or not ladies, we do not seek the same qualities in our work partners as we do in our wives or girlfriends. The reason is quite simple. Our wives and girlfriends are women we cherish as companions, roomies, and dates. We need a woman to have and to hold, to trust beyond measure; a friend we can always count on in good times and bad, just as they need the same from us. It would be great if our female co-workers had some of these traits, such as being trustworthy and good friends, but that's as far as our relationships can go. Of course I am speaking for the men that are already taken. Some single men may be looking for female co-workers with fringe benefits but that's another story entirely and not one that I care to exploit at this time. I was single for almost fifteen years while working as a sterile processing technician, so I know what it's like to be infatuated with female co-workers, and I've also dated a few. I don't see anything wrong with that and neither did anyone else, as long as we kept it on the down low and continued to prioritize our work as the most important reason we were there. Anyway, before I drift too far off the subject, for the most part men expect the same qualities in a female co-worker as they do in their male counterparts: dependability, helpfulness, a strong work ethic, and the ability to get the job done. Any woman who has three out of four of these traits at work will get kudos and compliments from the men on the job. Of course if a female co-worker is attractive that is an added bonus but it doesn't really matter in the scheme of a busy work day unless of course a man is single and looking.

Oh and one last thing while I have the ladies' attention. Men don't change a whole lot just because we are at work. Most guys just don't find it interesting to discuss shopping, furniture, or hair and nail appointments. So girls, if you are looking to chat with someone just for the sake of talking something out, please don't come to us with your female conversations. I'm sure it can wait until the next woman walks into the department from break. Just because we elected to work in a department noted for its prolific female population doesn't mean we've traded in our man cards for a box of chocolates or a dozen roses. Even wives know enough not to talk to their husbands about *everything*. Well you know what I mean. If I don't want to hear my wife ramble on about something, I surely don't want to hear about it from a woman I work with. But I'm not revealing anything most women don't already know.

So to close out this chapter on working together in sterile processing, I hope I've covered enough ground to at least break the ice between anyone new to the department and their fellow co-workers. I barely scratched the surface but psychology on the job can get pretty deep. I bet there have been entire books, even college courses, devoted to the subject. In fact, if you really want to dive into it wholeheartedly there are *master's degree* programs in occupational psychology. That's right; more commonly called **Industrial/ Organizational Psychology**, it is "the science of human behavior relating to work and applies psychological theories and principles to organizations and individuals in their places of work as well as the individual's work-life more generally." (Truxillo, D. M., Bauer, T. N., & Erdogan, B. (2016). Psychology and Work: Perspectives on Industrial and Organizational Psychology. New York: Psychology Press-Taylor & Francis.) So there you go. You can pursue a Master's of Science degree in I/O Psychology at just about any university in the U.S. and learn all about the art of getting along at work. Of course if you had an M.S. degree in Psychology you wouldn't be looking for a job as a tech in sterile processing, now would you?

5 DIFFERENT HOSPITALS, SAME ENVIRONMENT

No matter where you go in the United States it's comforting to know that the majority of hospitals look familiar on the inside. That's because they have a lot in common. Naturally there are differences, some of them major ones, but there are characteristics that all hospitals share, and this is why you always get that indescribable 'feeling' whenever you step foot into one. Some may call it reassuring while others get the creeps, but there is a definite feeling that this is no normal building you have just entered. There is something special about it. And it's true. There is something special about a hospital.

Think of all the different kinds of big buildings you have been in or might come across throughout your life. There are condominiums, hotels, office buildings, millionaires' mansions, department stores, shopping malls, and so on. Now, just like when you took Anatomy and Physiology, think of the *structure and function* of each building. I'll wait…..

There is likely no modern structure built for public use that rivals a hospital in daily operational costs and annual budget allowances for new equipment, employees, food, supplies, water, maintenance, and electricity. I've never read the financial reports or been on any budget committees at the hospitals where I worked but it doesn't take a genius to notice the ridiculous amount of monetary reserves needed to run an average sized medical facility. Think of the specialized departments: The pharmacy and all of the prescription drugs; Radiology and all the exorbitant X-ray equipment; Endoscopy and their flexible endoscopes; The surgical suite with their robotics, anesthesia machines, and scads of other equipment worth millions of dollars; Sterile Processing and all the equipment and machinery we've been discussing in this book; and all the nursing units in the rest of the hospital, each with their own med rooms, supply rooms, and patient rooms, which by the way are each supplied with *crazy expensive* beds, IV pumps, and bathrooms. It's mind boggling when you start thinking about it. Small wonder the cost of healthcare is all but unaffordable to those with anything but full coverage medical insurance.

And the *garbage*! If all the environmentalists in the world had the opportunity to spend a day at an average sized (say 350 beds) hospital in the U.S. they would likely form a huge rally to shut half of them down and force the other half to burn their own trash in on-site incinerators. When I see the amount of trash thrown away each day in our department alone I cringe. I can't even imagine why the oceans aren't already overflowing with medical waste. I don't know the answer but it doesn't take a mastermind to figure out the obvious.

There has got to be a better way to conserve our natural resources and save this planet from the inevitable. Making everything out of disposable plastic and throwing it away after each patient use doesn't seem to be the smartest thing to do. One hundred years from now I hope they will look back on this practice and scratch their heads wondering how the entire community of healthcare professionals and legislators could be so ignorant and irresponsible. But that is the status quo practice in hospitals today.

Another attribute that sets hospitals apart from other buildings is the health status of their occupants, which is assumed to be let's just say *not well*. There are a lot of sick people in a hospital; so many that it might seem they outnumber the healthy. The nurse-to-patient ratio might lead the lay person to believe that there are far more patients than medical staff on any given day. But think about the aforementioned specialized departments and all the staff it takes to run them. Then add the environmental services, nutritional services, and engineering departments and you can see why an average hospital's staff outnumbers its patients by a ratio of four to one. The data for this statistic is available in an article written by *Laura Dyrda* for the e-zine **Becker's Hospital Review** entitled "50 things to know about hospital staffing." According to the article, written in February 2017, hospitals with between 300 and 399 beds (which I have been calling average size) should have a full-time staff of roughly 1700. So yes, there are a lot of sick people in hospitals compared to say department stores or condominiums (at least one would hope). But realize that for each one of those sick people there are at least four relatively healthy people whose jobs in one way or another are going to affect the outcome of their stay. If you take nothing else away from these statistics, at least wrap your mind around the idea that it takes four people to care for one patient in the majority of today's hospitals. Is this a good thing? Well, if every healthcare worker in every facility is living by the creed "First, do no harm" then sure, why wouldn't you want as many people caring for the patient as is affordable. The more the merrier when it comes to caregivers, right? I suppose there are times when too many nurses or doctors might get in each other's way, such as in an operating room. For most surgeries it is preferred to operate with one doctor, perhaps his/her assistant, a surgical tech, the anesthesiologist, and the nurse. Anyone else in the room is presumed to be in the way or just an observer. The operating room would likely be considered an exception to the rule that more is better when it comes to medical staff. Anywhere else in the hospital I would say hire as many as the budget allows. Not enough help serving up food in the cafeteria? Hire someone. Is the trash piling up in the dirty holds? Hire more EVS workers. Is the OR constantly calling Central Service for trays that should have been sterilized an hour ago? Boy does this one hit home! Get some more sterile processing techs in there! Saving lives and healing the sick is what healthcare is supposed to be all about. Too many hospitals these days make it more about ensuring that the CEO's and upper management make it onto the Fortune 500 list. I'm not saying most hospitals are like that; on the contrary. I think there are more state-of-the-art healthcare facilities than ever before in the U.S. and around the world today. But ten 500-bed hospitals out of one thousand that care more about their image than their patients is ten too many. 'Nuff said about that. A lot of us who have worked at various facilities have either worked for or know about one like this. They will spare no expense to have the latest gadgets, promote the latest trends, or shove their latest slogan down your throat, but when it comes down to the moment of truth, do they deliver the goods? Only a hospital with good management and the right people can do that. The proof is in the pudding, as they used to say when I was growing up.

Yet another feature in every hospital is the Emergency Room, or as they are called more often today, Emergency Departments. Every hospital's got one; let's face it if it doesn't have one it's not really a hospital, is it? There is an old saying that the Central Service department is the "heart of the hospital."

Figuratively speaking that may be so. Without sterile supplies, bandages, sterile surgical instruments, and clean IV pumps, a hospital could not survive, nor could it save any patients. Yet I would submit that the *real* heart of every hospital is its Emergency Department. Walk down any hallway in a hospital and you will find an almost routine type of atmosphere. There are cafeteria workers carrying food trays into patient rooms; radiographers pushing portable x-ray machines around; lab workers drawing blood; EVS personnel mopping and cleaning rooms after each patient's discharge; doctors doing their rounds to check up on their patients, perhaps following surgery; and nurses answering their patients' "buzzers" or lights, however they've been instructed to communicate with them. Taking care of patients on the floors has taken on an almost routine nature. Any commotion coming from a particular patient's room is conspicuous and usually means that someone wants a higher dose of painkiller or whatever medicine he or she is taking. Otherwise an average day on the floors consists of hearing a lot of different TV sets playing everything from old **Gunsmoke** episodes to popular shows like **Dancing with the Stars**. Now head downstairs and take a walk through the Emergency Department, but try to stay out of the way. It's not uncommon to see nurses and E.D. personnel literally running from room to room to check on the status of unstable patients. And it is anything but quiet! You might hear babies crying, children screaming, grown men and women hollering for help, or all of the above at the same time. The Emergency Room's pulse never stops. But you don't have to take my word for it. Think about all your favorite hospital shows on television, from **St. Elsewhere** to **ER** and **Grey's Anatomy**. Whenever the scene switches from an intern shadowing a doctor on the floors to a code that has just been called in the E.R., suddenly everyone's heart rate goes up, from the nurse who called the code to the first responders and anyone else within earshot of the call, including the audience sitting in front of their TV sets in the comfort of their homes. The true heartbeat of the hospital never stops, and it is alive and pumping in the Emergency

Department.

Notwithstanding the plug for the E.D., I do understand why Central Service has long been known as "The Heart of the Hospital." As a metaphor, it is a perfect way to describe how all the life-sustaining supplies come from there and are transported throughout the rest of the hospital, just as blood is transported from the heart and flows through the body via the arteries and veins. Without Central Service there would be no supply depot, no in-house sterilization, and no way of reprocessing instruments for surgery. Another way of looking at it is a person without any 'heart' lacks the spirit, drive, and willpower to thrive in his or her environment. So too a hospital without a Central would not have the drive to make it through each day and therefore could not make it in today's busy environment.

So now that I've beat that to death, let's just say that the Emergency Department is the heart *beat* of the hospital. Maybe we can cover all the bases that way.

And since we were on the subject of all the hospital related programs that have ever been on television, do you suppose the drama depicted on those shows was based on reality? I'm not talking about drama with patients; we know that is real. What about the way those shows always assumed there was drama going on between doctors and nurses, nurses and patients, doctors and patients, doctors and other doctors and well, you get the point. Do you suppose that happens in real life? In my personal observations over the years I would say that yes it really does happen but, as in most every other situational drama on television, the producers tend to spend too much time on the behind-the-scenes personal relationships. Nurses really do fall for doctors and other nurses, just as a radiographer might fall for a physical therapist he or she happens to meet while shooting X-rays in a patient's room one day. That's just fate. As for those steamy scenes about secret rendezvous in empty patient rooms, supply closets, and any other opportunistic portals of privacy that allegedly abound within a hospital's premises, I can only repeat what I have heard. And the answer is still yes with the same caveat. Those risqué love scenes that would appear to be routine occurrences in every hospital in the country, according to television, probably don't happen quite as often as they would have us think. I'm not even going to guess at how the reality version compares to the fictionalized TV drama, but I do know there is a certain amount of professionalism expected of every employee while on the job, and if they cross the line and get caught one too many times their job will most likely be in jeopardy. And I have actually heard of that happening to at least one pair of risk-takers. They both worked in the same department and one was the other's department head. They were both married, not to each other, and had been "meeting" secretly for at least a couple of years before they got caught. In truth, many other employees around the hospital and in their own department knew about their rendezvous, but no one wanted to say anything because of the stature of the department head's position. They had both been prominent figures in their respective careers. When the truth finally became too much for the whole department to bear, they were both fired. Some of the stories that went around about how and where they would meet were every bit as dramatic as any top-rated daytime hospital drama. So the answer to that question is yes, that kind of stuff still goes on, but I would venture to say not as much as it used to. The clinical and professional attitude that dominates the scene in modern day hospitals makes risqué rendezvous less common and more risky than it was when shows like **General Hospital** and **Medical Center** romanticized the hospital culture for all it was worth.

Not that romance in a hospital setting always has to be a secret or a devious act worthy of a best-selling novel. There are also true stories of relationships born in the bustling daily routines of healthcare workers that rival any heartwarming Disney fairy tale. I've known several colleagues who have dated other techs they met on the job. Some of them worked in the same department while others just happened upon each other as they were going about their daily assignments. A few of my co-workers have even met the loves of their lives while working in the hospital. This should not be surprising to most people, as a hospital is a lot like a self-contained city within a building, much like a cruise ship, and we all know about the romances that blossom on a cruise ship. And no I'm not comparing the atmosphere in a hospital to *"The Love Boat"*; just saying it's not a bad place for singles to meet interesting people for friendship, dating, or even something more serious if that's what they are looking for. One of the more popular places to meet someone would be in the cafeteria, and this also should come as no surprise. Workers are off the clock, hence more relaxed and more likely to want to talk about something (or *anything*) other than work. One word of caution: If you are looking to get to know someone better while eating with them in the cafeteria, some of the larger hospitals can be pretty cliquish when it comes to lunch or dinner partners. Remember all through school when you would usually sit with the same group of kids each day that you sat with on the first day of school each year? Consider that once a healthcare worker decides who they are going to eat with every day it becomes almost ritualistic. Now consider this scenario: You meet a really nice tech over in the OR and she takes a liking to you, so you both agree to meet over lunch in the cafeteria, which she always takes at 12:30. You're getting all excited thinking about how awesome your lunch date is going to be, so you clock out at 12:20 and head down to grab something to eat. After paying for a hot dog and soda you head out into the lunch room and look for your luncheon partner. She is already sitting at a full table and waves you down. The closer you get to her table the more you realize she is sitting with all of her buddies from the OR. Some luncheon date, huh? But that's the reality in most of the larger hospitals. Because they are almost always situated in the middle of large metropolises with the inherent crime that goes along with the territory, cliques are often the norm, just like back in school. So you're going to notice a lot of same-colored uniforms at each table in the cafeteria. Anyway, if you decide to stick it out and her friends and co-workers like you, who knows? You may have just found a new partner. In any case, nothing ventured nothing gained as they say.

One last thing while we are on the subject of some of the similar features hospitals share; it coincides with the first paragraph in this chapter about some people getting the "creeps" when they step foot into one. Do you think some hospitals could be haunted? Some workers, mostly on the night shift, would swear to it. There are the usual claims of creaking stairs; footsteps heard walking down a hallway with no one there; voices coming from empty rooms; elevators going up and down with nobody inside, and endless other unexplainable phenomena often seen on television shows about ghostly sightings in creepy old haunted mansions. I confess that in thirty years of working in healthcare I have never seen any firsthand proof that hospitals are haunted. Yet I always gave a certain amount of credence to the stories heard along the way about the strange goings on that occur on the night shift. Why? Because there is definitely a spiritual world that none of us can explain to the fullest. Who is to say that hospitals could not be an outlet for spirits? Lord knows there are plenty of patients over the years that never make it out of there alive.

The spookiest building I've ever been in was an old hospital in North Carolina that had been converted into apartments. We were visiting a relative there who took us down an elevator to the basement, which had been vacant since the building was converted. There was a long long hallway that lead to nowhere, cobwebs everywhere; right out of **"The Twilight Zone."** I'm telling you, you couldn't pay me to take that elevator down to the basement in the middle of the night. Take a night watchman's job in that place? I don't think so.

Well that about does it for features that make hospitals the unique structures they are. Aside from all these features and a few I may have overlooked, each hospital has its own distinct footprint, if you will. Each one is managed differently, has its own blend of technology, and has its own unique history. One thing is for sure, just because you've seen one hospital does NOT mean you have seen them all.

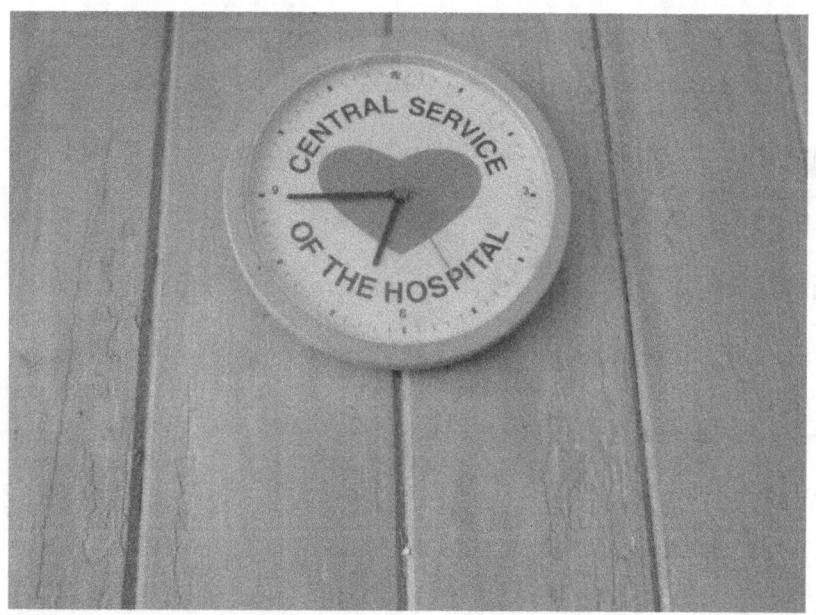

6 TEACHING STERILE PROCESSING IN A LARGE HOSPITAL

According to 20th century German-American psychologist Erik Erikson, there are eight stages of psychosocial development in life, assuming one lives to the wise old age of 65 and beyond. The seventh stage (ages 40-65 years) is the **Care: Generativity vs. Stagnation** stage. According to *Wikipedia*, Erikson himself coined the term "generativity." It is the "ability to transcend personal interests to provide care and concern for younger and older generations."

Many of us trudge through early adulthood with our 'noses to the grindstone' as the old saying goes, just trying to keep our heads above water to support ourselves and our families. There are very little time or extra resources for the average worker to play philanthropist or even think about helping the rest of society. There is however a light at the end of the tunnel for the diligent worker who has planned carefully and been able to actually keep his or her head above water throughout young adulthood. By the way, Erikson called this the first stage of adulthood (ages 20-39 years), or **Love: Intimacy vs. Isolation**.

What does all this have to do with sterile processing? I would be happy to explain. As you might already know if you are a tech, or you may have gathered if you've been paying attention, sterile processing is becoming more and more complex as technology advances by leaps and bounds day to day and year after year. Yet I doubt that as a career it will ever require more than a diploma at the most to land an entry level position in the field. And that is a good thing. It is probably one of the most technical jobs one can perform in a hospital without some kind of degree. It can be a wonderful career for someone who doesn't have the time or the resources to get a technical degree but enjoys being surrounded by new technology. Sterile processing technicians handle hundreds of thousands of dollars worth of instruments *each day*, and if you include the machinery those figures could easily jump into the millions. Of course when it comes to the technological hierarchy we are at the low end of the totem pole because we just handle the equipment; we don't actually build it or use it. Still, when there is that much of a department's budget tied up in instruments and equipment it helps to know how to handle it properly. And when there are patients involved, learning how to clean and sterilize each item is a must. And this is where education comes in. But who can and should educate for sterile processing? Not such a tough question. Or is it? Most teachers hold at least a Bachelor's degree these days; in fact it is required in most states. But would you like to guess how many sterile processing techs have a Bachelor's degree? My guess would be less than one percent. Okay so let's forego that criterion. What about requiring an educator to have at least five years of experience in sterile processing or surgical technology? That sounds more logical but how does a person with experience in cleaning and sterilizing instruments parlay that skill into a teaching job with no previous teaching experience? Is the employer then supposed to require both teaching AND sterile processing experience? And how large does a hospital have to be before it is even feasible to hire an educator. After all, most hospitals use the shadowing technique, where new employees simply watch experienced technicians perform their duties and learn a little more each day until they are let loose after their probationary periods are over. Generally speaking, only the larger hospitals, for example over 800 beds, even consider hiring an educator to teach new hires and keep their experienced employees up to date using in-services and other special presentations. Not such an easy question after all, was it? Well I've got a little bit of experience on the subject so let me share with you what I have learned about sterile processing education.

My stint as a sterile processing educator was a brief one. It started out with so much promise and optimism but within a year from my hire date I was worse off than when that journey began. At least back home in Vero Beach I always knew where my next paycheck was coming from. Living in a big city with no job was more than just a little scary. Thankfully everything worked out okay in the long run, and it looks like God provided the educator position as a means of getting me to finally move out of my hometown of forty-two years.

If you ever want to take a crash course in something, apply for a teaching job in that subject. You will learn more in a shorter amount of time than if you just took on a regular position. This can be taken as a general statement to include teaching math, English, social studies, etc. in any school from elementary through college. Taken in the context of this book however, it means that you will learn more in one year of teaching sterile processing than you would in ten years as a regular tech. How do you train to be a sterile processing educator? There is no formal training program that I am aware of. Ideally a rookie educator should learn from a mentor, which would mean that the educator's boss would have been a former educator. I have no idea how many sterile processing departments operate under this "ideal" condition, but that was how I learned to be an educator and it was definitely a crash course. So let me take you through what it's like to teach for just one year at a level one trauma hospital in the state of Florida.

The first thing you should know is a sterile processing educator is a lot farther up the ladder than most technicians realize. The only person in the department who holds a higher title is the sterile processing manager. I tell you this just in case you were under the impression that an educator is nothing more than a tech that gets to teach new hires and give monthly in-services to their co-workers. This is a high profile job. To say I was taken aback when my new manager told me everything that the job entailed would be like saying the rain in Florida is wet. Picture this: A sterile processing tech of 17 years from a small town hospital, making an hourly wage of $10.50/hour, accepts a job in one of the largest hospitals in the state of Florida, which also happens to have Trauma 1 classification. This means they have to accept **any** patient no matter what status; car accidents, gunshot wounds, attempted suicides, severe burns, you name it. There are only ten Trauma One centers in the state of Florida. Within the first month of this new educator's hire date he has been formally introduced, thanks to his new manager, to not only the entire Central Service staff from the top down, but to the entire OR staff as well. That includes staff in two sister hospitals a block away from the main campus. In each introduction the manager presented the former tech to nurse managers, department supervisors, and even her own manager, like this new educator was going to be something *really special*. She would say,

"Have you met our new educator?"

To which I would extend a hand to greet yet another

superior officer. They would treat me with immediate dignity and respect while I responded by treating them like foreign dignitaries. That's right, if you hadn't already guessed, that former tech from a small town was me. That first month as an educator was both a humbling experience and a huge ego booster; humbling because I met so many important medical personnel that had undoubtedly helped save countless lives in one of the few level one trauma centers in the state. And of course it was an ego booster because come on, whose self-esteem wouldn't skyrocket into the stratosphere after all those introductions? After the first month the newness began to wear off just a little but the job was still exciting and a joy to wake up for every morning. I was adjusting more each day to my status as an educator, and my manager was showing me the ropes, making sure I didn't make any big mistakes that would get me into trouble with the higher-ups or the doctors. She was a great mentor and always let me know how proud she was with my progress by giving me a big smile and saying,

"I see a lot of potential. You're going to be great."

Life was good.

After the third month the 90-day probationary period was over and it was time to get to work. I would find out just what the educator position was all about now. What I found out was that I was still exactly where I wanted to be, but it was not going to be as easy as it looked in those first three enchanting months. This job was going to take every bit of resourcefulness I could muster. It was just like my manager had explained early on; most people are task oriented in their work but an educator must strive to be a critical thinker. I had just graduated from UCF with a bachelor's degree in psychology the previous spring and was eager to try some strategies we learned in school. I would try to keep it fun while digging in and learning everything there was to know about teaching the craft of sterile processing to large groups of techs I was just getting to know. Mind you I've never been much of a people person so this would also be a growing experience, one that would hopefully somehow convert my mostly introverted personality into more of an extroverted one. So you can see there were quite a few challenges the new educator would have to overcome in order to be successful. The first one was learning to teach a class.

Don't be surprised if the educator at your hospital teaches a class on Central Service. If the facility is large enough or part of a larger system of hospitals, they might even get to teach in a designated classroom. I taught a class of new hires every Monday for eight hours straight with a half hour lunch break, just like a day's work except it was held in a special classroom on another campus. The curriculum was taken almost verbatim from IAHCSSM's *Central Service Technical Manual* and included slide presentations, CD-ROM videos projected from a laptop onto a big screen, and hours of lecture. Even if you've never taught a class before, the nervousness goes away after the first hour of lecture each week. If you feel really comfortable standing and talking to small groups of people it shouldn't be a problem at all. I always got butterflies and still do, prior to any event where I have to do some type of solo performance. That's probably a common thing with most people. You just grit your teeth and go for it and the butterflies disappear after a few minutes. If you don't get butterflies under any circumstances then you are one cool customer. Anyway after each course was completed, about ten weeks if I remember correctly, the students who passed all the weekly quizzes graduated, their work was sent in to IAHCSSM and they would receive their certifications. So it was an important course and also a mandatory one, as my hospital required techs to be certified within six months of their hire date. Teaching an eight hour class every week is hard work, especially if you are not used to teaching, but like you always hear teachers say, it is definitely a rewarding experience.

Another skill a new educator has to learn is how to conduct him or herself at large board meetings. Remember all those nurse managers, department heads, and supervisors I mentioned that you will meet during the first month after getting hired? Those same medical executive types meet at least once a month in the boardroom to discuss important issues like budgets, P & P (policy and procedure), new ideas, and anything else that someone at the table wants to discuss. In the short time I was there I never once spoke at a board meeting. As Abraham Lincoln has been credited with saying,

"Better to remain silent and be thought a fool than to speak and to remove all doubt."

I think it was during my first board meeting I decided not to speak unless spoken to. One of the nurse managers from the OR raised her hand for permission to speak, and then spewed out so many acronyms in her first statement I swear she must have used every letter in the alphabet at least twice. And to top it off several of the other managers nodded their heads in total agreement like they understood exactly what she was talking about. She lost me after *"We need to address the P&P of the new SMR and how they relate to the IFU for the AER's."*

There are board meetings to attend and classes to teach but the real work of the sterile processing educator, the bread and butter, is gathering up new information each day for the weekly department in-services. Some weeks there is such an overflow of new information provided by instrument vendors, OR nurse managers, and the department manager that it is difficult to condense it all into the allotted half hour or so each Friday (or whenever). Other weeks are spent researching material that hopefully your boss has never even thought of before, just to present something new and useful to the team. During one of those slower weeks I made up a poster board that showed the principles of steam sterilization using old black and white drawings and photos taken from an old book titled **"Principles and Methods of Sterilization in Health Sciences"** (Second Edition), by John J. Perkins. The team loved it and it was one of my favorite presentations.

If you teach at a progressive hospital you will never

lack for new technology that will have to be demonstrated and explained to the team. Surgical instrumentation and equipment is developing at warp speed these days and each surgery department needs at least one person who can keep up so they can relay the information to the men and women who need it to work with. Teaching is a special talent. Anyone who aspires to teach should not only enjoy being around people but also must feel comfortable being in the spotlight every day. The educator is expected to know everything there is to know about sterile processing and that is a huge expectation. One must consider him or herself a **professor** in the field and act accordingly. Knowing IAHCSSM's *Central Service Technical Manual* backwards and forward is not only a plus; it is a must. No student or even a tech should know more about instrumentation and sterilization than the educator. And these thoughts are not my own; they come from the strict philosophy of my former manager. She could make it known just by the look on her face that if you were weak in any subject pertaining to the department, you did not fulfill her expectations. At the same time if one of her techs showed occasional flashes of brilliance they were given big smiles and kudos, an indication that if the educator continued to reveal a less than stellar knowledge base, perhaps a brilliant tech could be next in line for the job. The lesson here is: Don't expect any employer loyalty or job security during your first year on the job as a sterile processing educator at a large facility. If nothing else it will be a wild and unpredictable ride. So at least try to enjoy it. Realize that if you eventually succeed you have made one heck of an accomplishment and can go anywhere in the country with this skill.

If everything in the previous paragraphs weren't enough, a sterile processing educator, as part of the management team in a large hospital, has to learn to play politics, otherwise known as *the game*. Unfortunately I can't give you any tips on this subject and the reason is two fold. First of all I never cared to learn anything about playing politics; it has something to do with the way I was raised and the desire to be like my father when I was a boy. He had been raised as a farm boy just like his father, and went on to be a hard worker for the rest of his life. Looks like I have done a pretty good job of following in his footsteps in that regard. Secondly, that is likely the biggest reason I didn't last longer than a year in this career; and if that is the case then I can live with it. After thirty years of working hard for everything I ever got for it, I couldn't adjust to sitting at a desk behind a computer for thirty hours a week. There is no shame in that. There were also a lot of issues going on between my manager and me that I just could not deal with, but they do not belong in this book, as I have decided to leave most of the drama out of it. Back to *the game*: If you never had to deal with office politics before and you really want to succeed in this career, I suggest taking a class or two on the subject, namely **Political Science 101**. I'm not joking or exaggerating about this. Hard core political skills are mandatory to succeed in this business. Simply put, if you don't learn how to deal with people every single day who have the power to chew you up and spit you out like a rotten egg, you will never survive. And that *is* the best advice I can give you on this subject.

That's about all I have to say about the challenging yet rewarding career of a sterile processing educator. I hope I have been helpful and didn't scare anyone off; that was not my intention. I could have skipped the subject entirely just because I did not succeed in the position, but I chose to write about it just because it can be such a great job under the right circumstances. Those would include having a great manager that will show you the ropes *and* support you every step of the way. As you have seen from reading about my experience, there are no guarantees and it is quite a bit riskier than the average sterile processing career. Are the rewards worth the cost in stress and less job security than that of a regular tech? I can't tell you that. If you are young and going through that magical phase of trying new things till you get it right, then go ahead and give this career a chance. If you have a four year degree, your odds are even better. Youth and knowledge will be your strengths that you can leverage anywhere you go. Blessings!

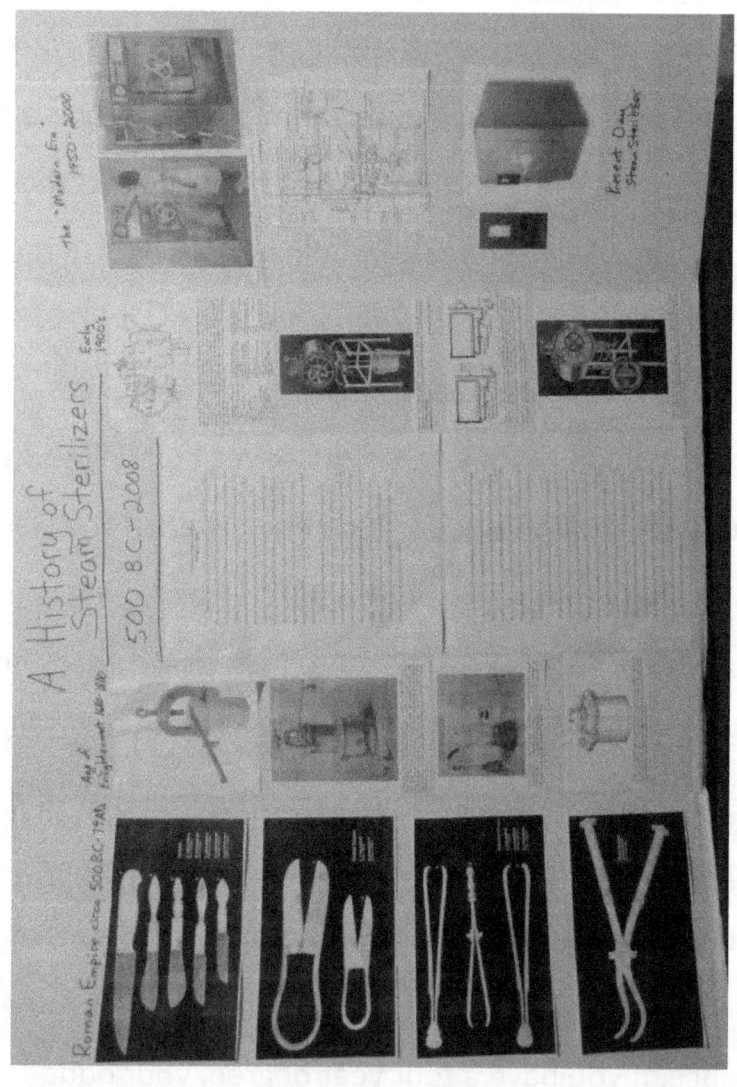

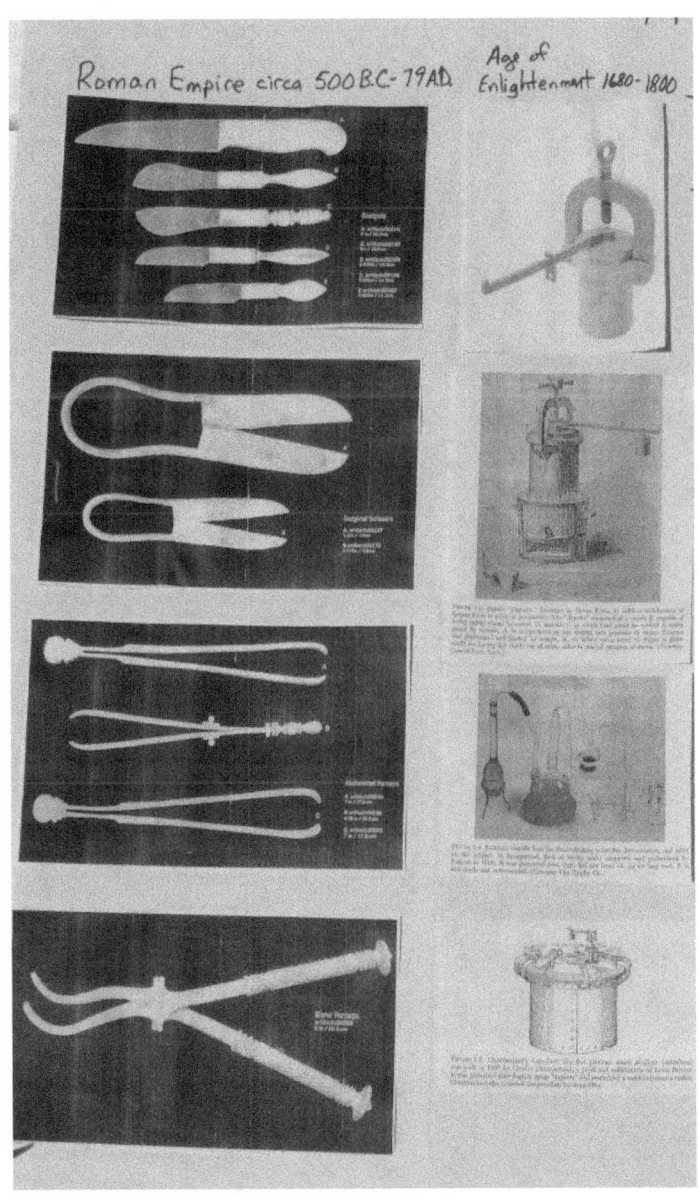

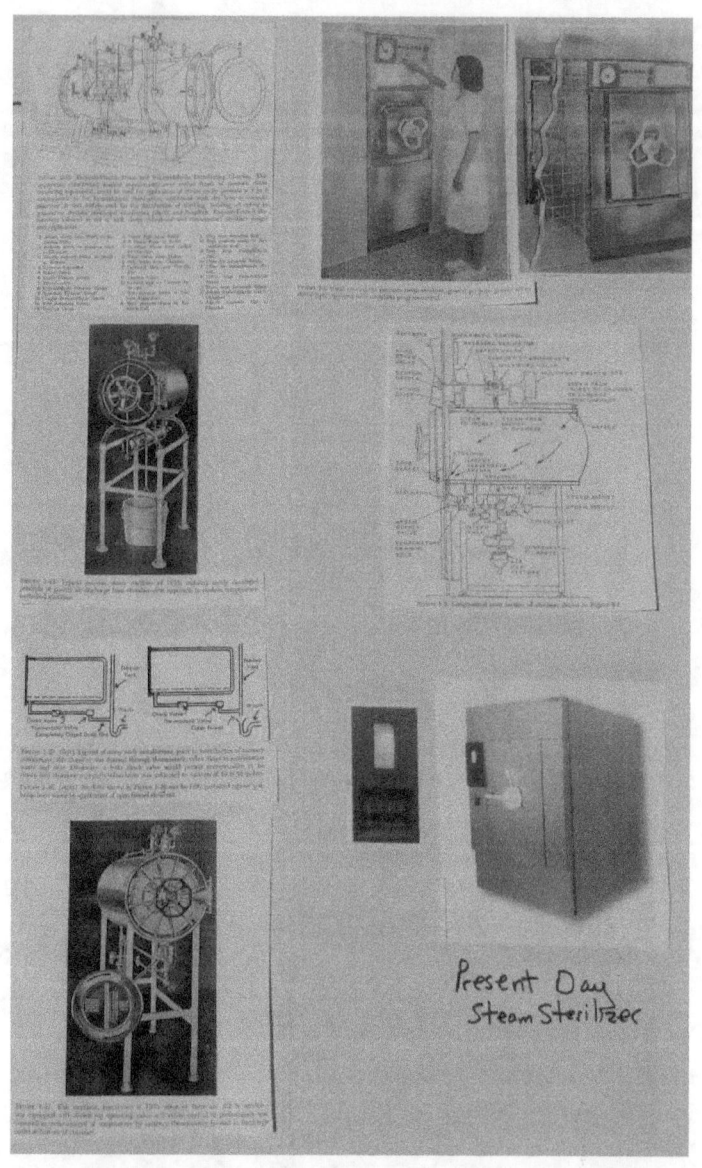

My presentation as an educator.

7 EXPERIENCE IS KEY

When I first sat down to write this chapter it seemed like a challenge to fill up more than a couple of pages stating the obvious, that "experience is key." I almost decided to nix it and move on to the next chapter. Chapter Eight's title, "Is there a Right Time to Move on?" sounded a lot more interesting and informative. But the writer's muse won out and so we will discuss the advantages of having years of experience in sterile processing.

Whether you've stuck with this career for twenty years or more because you really love it or you are stuck in this career because you don't know what else to do, you've got a lot of experience cleaning, sorting, assembling, wrapping, and sterilizing surgical instruments. And that is nothing to sneeze at anymore because believe it or not there are hospitals out there willing to pay sterile processing techs a decent wage for their rare talents; just wanted to put that out there. No longer does one have to work two jobs or practically live in poverty because he or she has decided on making a career out of this type of work. Starting pay is still quite low for uncertified, inexperienced techs but certification and experience should bring in a much more attractive salary after a few lean years.

Now someone who has never worked in a hospital and never has the desire to do so might argue that hospital workers should not be attracted to the potential of making money. Rather they should love their jobs and perform it out of the sheer kindness of their hearts. I have to refer these people to scripture, specifically *1 Timothy 6:10*, which states that the **love** of money is the root of all evil. In this context it means that if someone pursues a career in nursing, radiology, or respiratory therapy solely for the attractive salaries of these highly prized medical careers, they will not likely succeed, nor would they ever be satisfied. Yet to deny hospital workers, whatever their career, of making a comfortable living because they have chosen to make a difference in the lives of patients is not only unrealistic but also unfair.

From a psychological perspective, one of the problems of being an underpaid worker in general and sterile processing tech in particular, is that after awhile one believes his or her work has little value in the company, in this case a hospital. When a tech believes this he (or she) usually takes on one of two different attitudes. (1) The tech might become discouraged with hospital work overall, and decide that it just isn't his or her calling, or (2) One may look upon sterile processing as a good learning experience and use it as a starting point for another career in healthcare. The second attitude is more positive but in both cases the sterile processing department has lost another tech. This is exactly what happens and that is why experienced sterile processing techs are few and far between, certainly in some parts of the country more than others. And that is a shame because experienced techs are what this chapter is all about.

I once read a post on a social media page for sterile processing technicians. It was apparently written by a department manager who claimed she would rather hire an employee with little to no experience in Sterile than hire someone with a lot of experience. She did not go into further detail on that particular post but someone who followed her tweets on a regular basis might have figured out her reasons for such a peculiar statement. I believe the discussion pertained to the cleaning of certain instruments in decontam and following the IFU's. If I may interject my thoughts on why someone would hire a green employee over an experienced one; the word is **stubborn** and it runs rampant among those of us with over ten years of experience in this field. Anyone with over twenty years – forget it! Part of the reason is that when we came up through the ranks during our first few years as techs, IFU's were not the exclusive rules to follow during our daily assignments. Back then we were allowed to use a little more common sense and we also followed whatever protocols our supervisors had laid out for us. Nowadays it's like I said, forget about it. Your supervisor isn't even allowed to have an opinion about the best way to clean an instrument, and if you so much as mention the words 'common sense' when asked why you did what you did, it could mean a trip to the office or worst case scenario, a write-up. In some hospitals this could be a slight exaggeration but in a lot more it is spot on. Seriously, the only acceptable answer would be "I was only following the IFU's."

There are many other examples of stubbornness in the workplace (I'm sure that manager on social media could come up with a whole slew of them). There is the matter of the interpretation of "fairness" by experienced workers vs. inexperienced workers vs. management. For instance, in one hospital I worked at we were expected to clean all the I.V. pumps that were brought down from the floors each day. It's one of those jobs that have to be done but nobody likes to do it. Everybody in our department had to accept that they were going to clean pumps every now and then. The majority of our experienced workers felt that after a certain amount of accumulated time on the job one should not have to clean pumps [that much] anymore. The feeling was that it should be a job for rookies and part-time help. The new workers, on the other hand, hated cleaning them because they felt the money they were being paid wasn't enough to compensate for the amount of misery involved in cleaning pumps. The management of course wanted everyone to do their part *equally* because they felt that was the only way to split up the job fairly. They also felt that the experienced workers should not have any complaints about doing any job asked of them because they were making more money than the new hires and therefore should be willing to do anything. And so it went.

Another complaint managers have about techs with experience, especially from other facilities, is that they tend to hold onto their old ways of doing things. Supervisors get tired of hearing about how things were done at your last hospital. I once knew a tech that talked about how they did things where he used to work almost *every single day*. It is okay to reminisce about your old jobs every now and then, and human nature to get homesick too; but try not to overdo it. Starting a new job is similar to moving to another country. Your newly adopted country is not going to change everything just to accommodate your old habits and cultural differences. Sooner or later you will have to *assimilate* to your new surroundings. Like everything else this is easier for some than it is for others.

Probably the most convincing reason for managers to shy away from experienced sterile processing techs (SPT's) is that some of them take shortcuts in both the decontaminating and assembly phases of the job. In the eyes of an SP manager or supervisor that is taboo with a capital **T**. It goes against everything that is preached to techs since our first day on the job. Remember: *Primum non nocere* – First do no harm. It's the reason we are taught to follow the manufacturers' IFU's to the letter whenever we wash and disinfect or sterilize any medical device. And with the ever-present threat of lawsuits and/or failed inspections by The Joint Commission that could close a hospital down with the stroke of a pen, it's no small wonder a manager would steer clear from SPT's with a resume boasting of **"Over 15 years of experience in Sterile Processing."** And yet for all the precautions taken to protect the patient, the situation is no different than in any other career. Experienced employees learn to take shortcuts. It's not only human nature; sometimes it is necessary, I mean let's face it. Budgets are cut and the number of employees is kept to a bare minimum during hard times just to keep a company afloat. It applies to almost every type of business across the board; the auto industry, the airlines (Remember the air traffic controller crisis of the 1980's?), agriculture, transportation; the list goes on and on. Employees are forced to do their jobs with a bare minimum of help from other co-workers. It is during these trying times that many of them learn to take shortcuts in order to get the work done. Weeks of working shorthanded can turn into months and even years. Meanwhile the shortcuts those employees have learned become their new routines. The supervisors may talk about them as if they are criminals but these hard working employees learned their 'poor habits' through necessity during hard times and with little help from their supervisors.

The argument for hiring inexperienced techs is a strong one. They can be shown exactly how they are expected to do their job, and have no knowledge of any other way the job can be done. In effect the company's way becomes their way. More specifically, the *supervisor's* way becomes their way. And the supervisors are under so much pressure in the current hospital setting to follow IFU's that it all comes back around to following IFU's. So if a sterile processing department is staffed with workers who instinctively follow the

manufacturers' Instructions for Use it makes
management's job a whole lot easier, at least in theory.

A problem with that theory is that if you purposely
staff a department full of inexperienced techs simply for
the sake of having no one there with previous
knowledge on the subject, well that is exactly what you
will have. It is what it is. The desire for having employees
who know of no other way to do their jobs except how
they were shown at their present facility is just slightly
short of being ignorant. And ignorance, though blissful,
is no way to run a business, much less a department in a
hospital. When it comes down to whether you want a
department full of competent workers or just a bunch of
puppets who do whatever you tell them to do, in this
writer's opinion the old cliché "There is no substitute for
experience" rings true. I'm not saying don't hire new
people fresh out of school or fresh from another career;
heck, that's how all of us started out. All I'm saying is
there is a definite need for experienced workers in every
sterile processing department. And they should get a

chance to speak their minds, whether it is their own opinion or to say that their last hospital did something a little differently. We can all learn from each other and that means other facilities too. As long as everyone keeps an open mind and doesn't dismiss anyone else's ideas just because they are not their own, we can each contribute something every day at the workplace. And that goes for both experienced and inexperienced workers. It even applies to the new employee who just left a career in the restaurant business to start a new one in the hospital. He or she might have some unique and impressive ideas about how to organize a decontam room after five years of experience in a gourmet kitchen. Don't laugh; a well organized kitchen in a large gourmet restaurant may be heads and tails above what you might encounter in many a hospital's decontam. In fact, a couple of the best sterile processing techs I have ever known were hired after transferring from our own hospital's cafeteria. It's kind of like when I first started in this line of work and all the linen, towel packs, biological test packs, and virtually everything else was reusable instead of disposable. Back then if you had a lot of experience folding and packing linen you were ready for a job in sterile processing. Workers who transferred from the hospital's laundry department found it a smooth transition. Today, with more and more hospitals going digital, perhaps the best experience one can get to prepare for a job in the medical field is to learn their own laptop inside and out. The learning curve for the computer software used in today's sterile processing departments is steeper than perhaps any other facet of the job. Everything else can be learned by hands-on teaching methods, but if you are not computer savvy, some of the new software can be downright frustrating to say the least. So you can see how experience from other careers, as well as other SP departments from different hospitals, can be a big help in rounding out a good strong team of SPT's.

Now that I have made the case that experience is a valuable tool to have at one's disposal in any workplace, including an SP department, do you suppose there is an

optimum amount of experience to look for in an
employee in this field? Well I think I stated it in an
earlier chapter but in case I haven't, I am not a former
human resources worker or manager, nor have I ever
worked in the job counseling field. But as I have said, I
do have thirty years of experience in Central Service, and
25 of those years have been in sterile processing, so I
know a thing or two about experience in the profession.
As far as how much experience would be optimal in this
field, it would be silly to put a cap on it; that would just
defy everything I've just related to you about the
benefits of having experienced employees. I mean how
ridiculous would that be? But I will say this. There is a
significant amount of burnout in this career that can
occur anytime after ten years on the job without
changing shifts, departments, or hospitals. It could occur
sooner or it might occur later, depending upon the
individual's personality and his or her ability to
persevere. As I said earlier, this job does not change a
whole lot over the years. Technology changes of course,
and with that come certain *adjustments* the employee

must make to keep up with the daily assignments. But decontamination, assembly, and sterilization will always be the three facets of this job, at least well into the 21st century. What happens in the next century is anyone's guess, things are moving so fast now. Combine *job experience* burnout with *work experience* burnout and you have a recipe for a disgruntled employee who could definitely have a negative impact on the department's mental health and other employees' overall outlook on their daily activities. What does this mean? All it means is that if you have a senior employee on the crew with over forty years of experience in the workforce and perhaps twenty of those years working in sterile processing, you've got someone who's probably not going to be very receptive to suggestions, change, or criticism; in short, all the usual feedback that employees experience every day on the job from their superiors. This is another instance that managers use to explain why they won't hire senior workers with a lot of experience. Have I already mentioned the word **stubborn**? So if you ever find yourself in the position of that senior citizen with a lot of experience, here is a tip to remember while you are shaking your head in frustration over the nonsense going on in your department: *Stay calm*. It's a simple message I know, and it might not even help out that much in removing your frustration, but like it or not you are your department's link to the older generation. If you act childish, moody, selfish, mean and stubborn, how do we justify telling the younger generation that they have no idea how hard we have worked throughout our lives? All they see is someone as old as their parents, aunts and uncles who can't even handle a normal day working in a hospital. I know it can be difficult but keep your negative thoughts to yourself for everyone's sake. Better still, so you won't hold onto those negative thoughts and get an ulcer, get rid of them. It is positive thinking that will see you through the tough times, days when you wished you didn't have to come to work every day; those days that make you long even more for retirement to hurry up and get here. For more about the power of positive thinking be sure and read through the entire last chapter of this book, for I intend to talk more about it in "God and Work."

I hope this chapter has served its purpose, and that was to show both sides of the coin in the argument over the need for experienced workers in sterile processing departments. In order to appreciate each other in a department that is bound to have workers from every level of experience, it is important to understand how each other feels. A key point is this: The experienced worker knows how the inexperienced worker must feel; he or she has been there before. The inexperienced worker knows little about how the experienced worker feels in this job. So there you have it. Compassion is the key.

8 IS THERE A RIGHT TIME TO MOVE ON?

It's not uncommon to leave a job after only a few months or even a couple of years when things don't turn out quite the way they were supposed to. Maybe the boss was let's just say a lot more personable and accommodating during the job interview than he or she turned out to be on a daily basis. Or perhaps the job itself started out okay but went downhill in a hurry. Maybe you don't get along too well with your co-workers. Could be the volume of work has almost doubled since you started and just getting busier. All these things can and do happen in almost any job and sterile processing is certainly no exception.

But what about the lifers? What about the workers who hung in there when layoffs were threatening to cut jobs, or when mandatory overtime forced everyone in the department to work 50 or more hours a week? How about the techs who report to work daily no matter if the air conditioner breaks down (happens all the time), half the equipment isn't working properly (sound familiar?), or most of the department is sick with the flu? What about sterile processing techs who have put in twenty or even thirty years in the same career, some of them in the same hospital? Is there ever a right time to leave this career or a sign that it is time to move on?

Of course you know the quick answer is that everyone's situation is different so there can be no standard one-size-fits-all solution. But let's go a little deeper and see if we can find any indications whatsoever that it is time to move on to another career. To many of you who have just started in your sterile processing career this chapter might seem meaningless. You may even want to skip it and that's fine. But to those few rare folks who have spent half their lives or more in this profession, I guarantee the subject is not meaningless. It is an important one and here's why. If you are at least 50 years old, that clock keeps ticking and you know what I'm talking about. If you have been in the same career, perhaps even in the same hospital for at least 20 years you've probably been wondering for quite some time now if there is something better out there. And with only 15 or so years of employment left it's time to either put up or shut up. Stay put or make a move. What are you waiting for?

I had a co-worker, a wonderful lady with whom I worked for several years. She had worked in sterile processing longer than I had, having started shortly after graduating high school. She had also been working at the same hospital for over twenty years in the same department. Like many techs who work in this field that long, she'd seen many changes. In fact the entire department had been rebuilt from what had been the old operating room prior to its reconstruction. Naturally the question would come up every now and then of whether she ever planned to leave the hospital or if she would retire there. Her position never changed. She would always say,

"I'm waiting for God to tell me when to leave."

Now I believe in God just as much as she does. If you believe in God no one can say to you, 'Well I believe in God more than you do.' It is true that some people have more *faith* in God than others, but if you believe then you believe and no one can take that away from you. I suppose if she has faith that someday God will move her from her position in sterile processing then it will surely happen but how will she know? What kind of sign is she looking for? I have asked her that question time and again and she does not know how God will tell her to move, *He just will.*

There may be others who share the same belief as my co-worker, and that is perfectly okay. In this writer's humble opinion, *It's better to believe in God and not know when or how He is going to move you than to not believe and think you know exactly what you are doing.* For the rest of you looking for logical answers to the question of how you would know if or when it is time to leave, let's take a look at some possible scenarios.

Scenario #1: A change in management. Most of us that have been working at any job for at least ten years have experienced this one. You've been trained to do every task exactly how your manager or supervisor wants it done. He or she knows you will do your job and do it well without much coaxing or prodding so you spend most of your typical work day basically unsupervised, just how you like it. Years go by with only the slightest hint of change because the boss man (or woman) has his or her own ideas about how to run the department and seldom waivers from the status quo. And then one day the inevitable happens. The supervisor or manager retires, quits, or is fired (I've seen all three), and all of a sudden the crew is left like sheep without a shepherd. They wonder, individually and collectively, what will become of them. Will the new supervisor or manager inconspicuously and methodically "let people go" in order to make room for his or her people? Many of us have seen that before. That would of course be the worst case scenario, especially if you really wanted to keep your job. But not to worry; it doesn't always happen that way. Sometimes the changing of the guard is totally favorable to existing employees and the new boss just wants a seamless transition from the old to the new, at least at first. Once they are settled in however, as Cyndi Lauper has sung, their "True Colors" will shine through, and there could be some major changes. Whether you feel ready to hang on for the ride or would much rather get off and try your luck at a different venue is totally up to you. Depending upon your circumstances it's usually more prudent to hang in there for awhile and try to be more open to change than was necessary in the past. Having said that, nobody can walk in your shoes and tell you how this new change will affect you in the long run. It's one of those gut things and you just have to trust your own instincts. I've had bosses before that I never thought I would be able to deal with on a daily basis for more than a few months at the most. And you know what? A couple of them turned out to be two of the most respectful and supportive bosses I have ever had. They were still difficult to work for at times, very demanding, but they respected me as a worker and because of that we understood what we had to do for each other. So just because a new boss might be difficult to get along with and you are two very different people, it does not mean you will not be able to work together. It only means at least one of you is going to have to try harder and it will most likely be you. So that's it for *scenario #1*. In a nutshell: Give new management a little time. They are just as uncomfortable as you with their new position. If after a year you still don't like the new direction they are going, and your comfort factor is declining exponentially with each passing week, then you might consider looking elsewhere for a better fit. Life is too short to spend your days in a job or career that makes you miserable.

Scenario #2: Burnout; plain and simple. It can happen in as little as a couple of years but usually a nice long vacation can cure that. I'm talking about the kind of burnout that starts around the seven-year-itch point in your career and spreads like a bad cold throughout your body over the next few years. The ten year mark in one's sterile processing career can make or break you and determine whether or not you will decide to stay put or move on. Oftentimes there has to be something to reach for, perhaps a higher level of certification; a really good reason to keep plugging away at the same job for another few years. Some people live their lives one day at a time; some live five years at a time. Almost nobody plans ten years down the road anymore except maybe those going after a professional degree. Life just seems to happen so fast these days that no one knows what it will be like ten years from now. I was scrolling through a social media page a couple of days ago and couldn't believe my eyes what I saw on a post from a golf course industry company. They posted a video of a totally autonomous fairway unit, basically a robotic mower without a driver. It was rolling down a fairway spewing grass out of the back of its reels like a boss. Now this might be old news to some of you who keep up with the latest technology but I was thoroughly blown away by that little video. In all of the ten years or better of working on golf courses in my younger days I don't think any of my co-workers or I ever envisioned that one day an entire golf course could be maintained by a bunch of robots. We watched Star Trek, sure, and some of us had also seen the movie "2001: A Space Odyssey" featuring HAL the robot who tried to take over a space ship. We all figured that someday NASA would land some type of robot on the moon or Mars or some other planet to take soil samples or perform some other mundane task that robots specialized in. But we never dreamed that golf course mowers would ever be able to drive themselves, especially the giant fairway units that required total concentration to operate inside of the perimeter of the fairways. My point is that nobody dares to wonder what life will be like ten years from now. Technology is moving too fast, and that includes the healthcare industry. Yet I digress. It's difficult to tell which direction we are headed into the future. I checked out one of those websites that try to advise people on which career to choose by judging the top twenty career choices for the next ten years. Their results: a full 80% were computer related; computer programming, computer engineering, computer repair, computer this, computer that, well you get the point. This is great news for those who always knew they wanted a career that involves computers. For the rest of us it doesn't leave a whole lot to the imagination. But seriously, getting back to *scenario #2*, if you do suffer from job burnout after only ten years in sterile processing, by all means take a break, especially if you are still young. Try something different; spread your wings. For your own good, don't make your whole life revolve around what happens between the walls of a sterile processing department. Life is too short and it will fly by before your very eyes unless you try different things. Our manager used to print out our work schedules in six-week increments so that there were only eight schedules for each year. I swear to you there is nothing that makes a year go by faster than watching your work schedules come and go. For those who have pets, it's worse than watching your puppy turn into an old dog in no time flat. Listen, if after you've played the field for awhile and seen what else is out there, you somehow miss the security of your old hospital job you can always find another one. Like I said before, thanks in part to our friend modern technology, sterile processing jobs abound in almost every part of the country. About the only reason you still never see it in the top twenty careers for the future is that the pay is still somewhat meager for all the skills and hardships involved. When and if they finally raise the average pay to a level equal to other semi-skilled jobs, you will start to see a dramatic increase in the exposure and popularity of our chosen career. Until then it will probably remain a **hidden culture**.

Scenario #3: Either you know too much or you just *think* you know too much. This is another one of those situations that can occur after the ten-year mark in one's career. Depending on one's personality it could occur a lot sooner but ten years seems to be a good benchmark for *scenarios #2 and #3*. It is around that time when the combination of burnout and **thinking you know all there is to know** can get you in trouble with your boss, manager, and other superiors. I think you might know what I'm talking about. There is an attitude that grows on a person after he or she has been doing the same job for a few years and doing it well. It comes with experience and coincides with what we were dealing with in the previous chapter *'Experience is Key.'* Simply put, people who have ten years or more experience are difficult to train when they have the attitude that there is nothing they can learn from anyone about their job. Looking at this problem from the employee's point of view can be just as frustrating. It can be very difficult to take instructions from someone with less time on the job or less experience in the field. Even worse is when the person instructing or giving orders does not seem to know what they are doing because of inexperience or lack of knowledge. This almost always causes friction between the worker and his or her superior and can lead to stressful working conditions for both. And we all know who is going to lose in that situation. A supervisor or manager can make life miserable for any subordinate who is uncooperative or unwilling to follow instructions. In a hospital these days, those instructions are often required to be followed to the letter. A simple example of *scenario #3* would be: say you've been wrapping trays using the **envelope technique** for over fifteen years. In my case it's been almost thirty years but let's say fifteen. A new supervisor comes onboard and says that the hospital where she came from uses the **square fold** method for wrapping. In an argument about which wrapping technique you should be using from now on, who do you think will win? My money is on the new supervisor. Better start practicing. For those who insist they really do know as much or more than their superiors about sterile processing, maybe it's time to put your money where your mouth is. You can talk the talk but can you walk the walk? Realize that in the eyes of management, anyone in a supervisory role is worth at least two, maybe three regular FTE's or techs. So if you can't beat 'em and you don't want to join 'em you know what the other alternatives are. Learn to get along or it might be time to hit the road. No need to fill your head with all kinds of scenarios and drama. There are only so many choices. In this case it's get off your high horse, learn to cooperate, and in time others including your superiors will automatically see that you do know your stuff. But it will never happen by continually getting into arguments with your supervisor, educator, or manager. Wait it out.

In all three scenarios you should note that the age of an employee who is on the verge of turning in his or her resignation plays an important role in the final decision. We've discussed this before but if you are young you should have a lot more flexibility in your choices, as opposed to if you are over 60. Once you start pushing that 60 year-old envelope there is a tendency to try to ride it out no matter how tough the going gets. Senior workers know all the old motivational mottos to keep us on track, such as "When the going gets tough the tough get going" or "Tough times never last, but tough people do." And once you're over what the Social Security Administration deems your **full retirement** age it gets harder each day to put up with all the politics and nonsense that are part of the daily work routine in a hospital. So as a general rule of thumb, if you're still young enough to move onward and upward as the need arises, by all means don't let anything or anyone stop you. If you've been hunkered down in the same place for awhile and it would be more difficult to pick up stakes than to stay put in your "miserable" job then here's what you do: make a list of all the positives and negatives of staying where you are and compare that to a list of the positives and negatives of moving to another job and then just weigh the results. Discuss everything with your spouse or significant other before making any final decisions and you're golden. No matter what your decision is remember there are no guarantees that everything will turn out peachy no matter where you end up. A pre-requisite to finding happiness in any job is contingent on having already graduated from the school of hard knocks. Successful completion of that school and a lot of prayer will get you through just about anything life throws at you.

There is an old saying I once saw on a bumper sticker back in the 1980's when bumper stickers were a lot more common than they are today. It read, "**Lead, follow, or *Get out of the way!*"** I never forgot that; it's not a bad motto for teamwork. A successful team requires good leadership and cooperation amongst its members. That doesn't necessarily mean that workers should follow their leaders blindly without even thinking about what they are doing. Be smart about it. It just means that if you know you've got good leadership then strive to be an important part of that successful team. If you are a strong leader then step into that leadership role when given the opportunity. If you can't do either one without causing a lot of friction and instability for the whole team then maybe you should try to find a job that is a better fit. Lead, follow, or get out of the way.

9 STERILE PREP TIMES

Since grade school I have enjoyed writing. In fifth grade our teacher had one particular writing assignment each Friday. She would pick the subject and we would have to write a short story about it. Most of the class dreaded the thought of making up a story and putting it down on paper but I didn't. One Friday the assignment was to create a mini mystery, sort of a spooky story; perhaps it was around Halloween. When she handed the papers back to us the following week there were comments written all over the two pages I had turned in. Afraid to read them at first, my fears subsided when I noticed the big red **A+** on the back page. The comments were all positive and the teacher was impressed. In those days I never reread anything after writing it down, so the first draft always sufficed. When I went back and read the scary mini-mystery written the previous Friday I was actually a little surprised and impressed as well, having no idea how the story turned out as scary or mysterious as it did. It was as if my imagination had totally overtaken the pen as I was writing.

These days my writing doesn't surprise me much anymore, or anyone else for that matter. You see I never pursued a career in writing so the skill never really blossomed. Pursuing a Bachelors degree in my forties rekindled the writing spirit (Gordon rule papers and Psychology research papers took care of that), and after graduating college I was eager to write something to prove that a Bachelors degree in Psychology is more than just a fancy looking piece of paper mounted in an overpriced and oversized frame. The first result was a newsletter printed and published by this author while working weekends at the hospital. After getting permission from the nurse manager I set out to write a monthly newsletter featuring articles of interest mostly about our sterile processing department. It started out slow; the first issue wasn't even two full pages, but it grew into something that after the fourth or fifth issue I was very proud of. After publishing about seven copies of each issue I would distribute them to various other departments, keeping two issues for our department, which we called "Sterile Prep." Here then, reproduced for your very own enjoyment and hopefully enrichment, are excerpts from the six original issues of "Sterile Prep Times", edited at my own discretion wherever there might be a violation of someone's personal or corporate rights.

I do have one request. For the 2nd Edition my wife and I both worked hard to ensure that the quality of the copies of "The Times" would be a significant improvement over the original book's version. Also, I have omitted several pages from the first edition that upon close scrutiny probably should not have been in there. Now here is the favor I ask of my readers: If anyone feels that certain content in this chapter should be omitted, please send your comments to my Amazon Author Page: amazon.com/author/hughesrick. In fact if you have any comments whatsoever, positive or negative, about this book as whole, I would like to hear them. You can also comment on and rate this book on its sales page on Amazon.com. Thanks and I would greatly appreciate that.

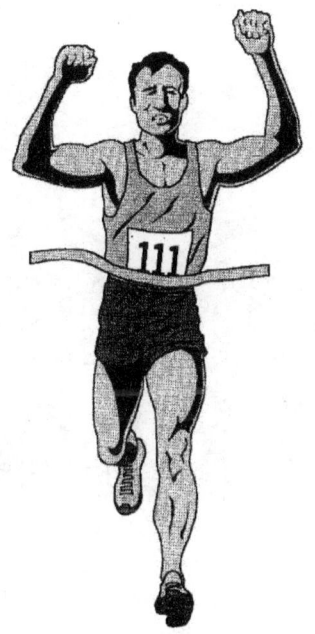

Hey, Gang!

It's the 1st issue of the brand-new in-house publication,

Sterile Prep Times.

The newsletter that dares to ask AND answer all of your questions about that most obscure of departments, Sterile Prep. Grab your souvenir copy today.

Picture From The Past

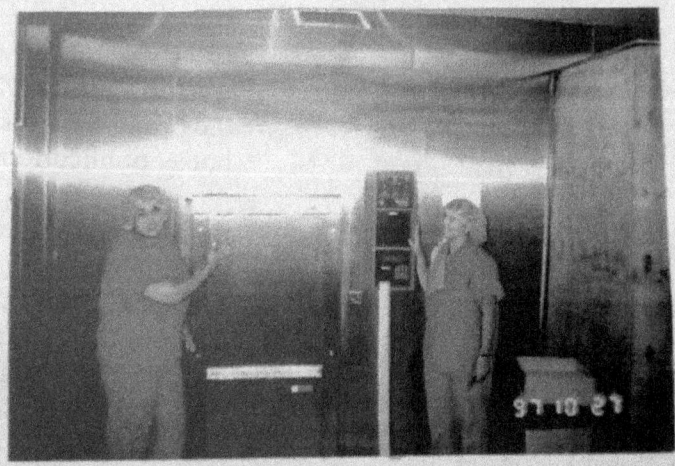

This picture, taken in October of 1997, shows two of our former Sterile Prep co-workers, Kathy and Taffy, showing off the brand-new autoclave steam sterilizers. The entire department was rejuvenated that year, and many of us who had worked awhile in the old department really appreciated the difference.

Until Next Time...

Thanks for reading our little newsletter. It has been a pleasure introducing you all to our department. Next month we will take a look at some of the instruments we clean and sterilize, and point out some of the areas where blood and other contaminants like to hide. See ya.

The Sterile Prep Times
Volume 2
May, 2004

Hi, friends and fellow workers. Here's hoping that your Spring is going well, and that you are preparing for the inevitable Summer, which will be here before you know it. Sterile Prep has had their hands full since the Winter months, keeping the Operating Room stocked with fresh instruments to accommodate all of our local patients, as well as our winter residents. Got to keep those snow birds happy, so that when they get back home they can brag about how smooth everything went

This is the second issue of *Sterile Prep Times*, one which I am sure you will find at least as enjoyable and informative as the first, which was distributed to five departments in the hospital that serve and/or are served by Sterile Prep. Last month I tried to familiarize you, our neighbors, with our friendly little outpost in the middle of the ground floor of our building. Recall that you made it all the way across the yellow line if you were in a pair of scrubs.

The Sterile Prep Times

3rd Edition

June 2004

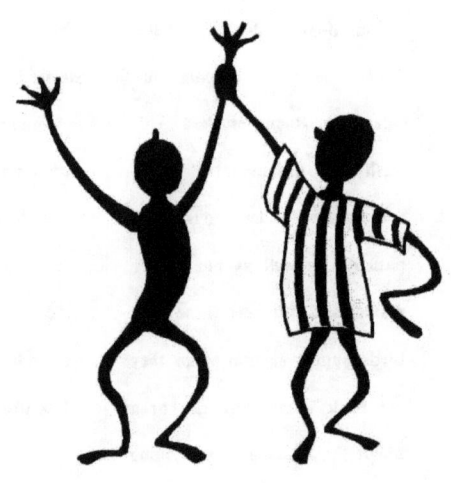

Long Ago, But Not Far Away

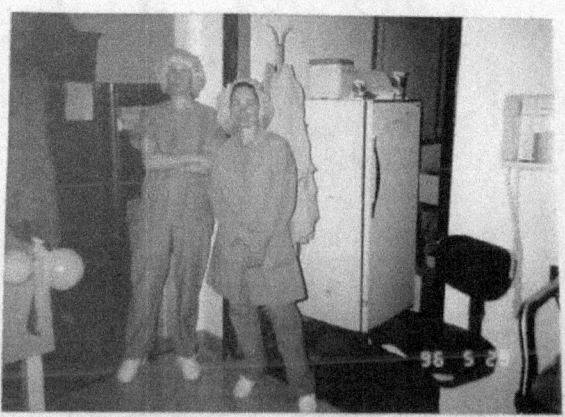

Here's a picture from the archives, of Linda and Sheila, two of our co-workers who are still with us, and still work together as a team. Eric, who now works in Special Procedures, looks on. The attire hasn't changed much in the past 8 years, although we are no longer required to wear the lab coat (such as the one Linda is wearing) whenever we leave the department.

Well, hey, gotta go. Hope you enjoyed this issue of The Sterile Prep Times. I look forward to the 4th Edition, when you can meet yet another one of our friendly staff, and we'll take a closer look at the *art* of sterilization. It'll be fun, so don't miss it! See ya.

The Sterile Prep
Times

4th Edition

July 2004

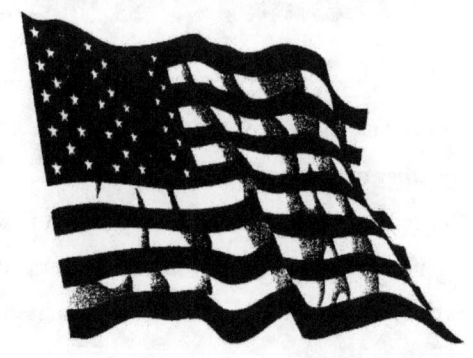

The Sterile Prep Times

4th Edition   July 2004

Greetings, all. Welcome to the 4th issue of SPT. Hope your summer is being filled with the titillating aroma of something tasty cooking on the grill. Time to round everybody up and head down to the beach, or the river, or the pool, or just find a huge shade tree and have yourself a picnic. You all know the drill: STAY COOL.

Anyway, I think I've thrown a really good paper together for you this month, hopefully one that is both informative and entertaining. Along with the regular departments that are fast becoming the SPT standard (OR Links, Employee intro, and a Picture from the past), there is a semi-in-depth article entitled "The Art of Sterilization" which conveys the actual process we go through minute by minute, every day, ad infinitum. Through the use of pictures and step-by-step descriptions, you will see how we clean, wrap, and sterilize the doctors' instruments following every surgery. Since this is a family oriented newspaper, there are no photos of the instruments as they would appear right after surgery, so I will simply tell you that the techs have their work cut out for them in decontam, where the process begins.

If that weren't enough, I am adding a new column in this issue called, "How does that work?" designed to show you, the reader, how some of the most advanced instruments in the operating room today make the job at hand much easier for the doctor, and thus better for the patient. ENJOY!

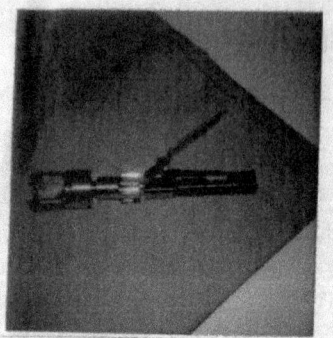

How Does it Work?

As a method of capturing the readers' interests and broadening everyone's horizons, as well, I am introducing a new segment to the regular format this month. This column will seek out the latest in surgical instrument technology and attempt to explain the function of each new device.

The first tool in our arsenal that we will take a look at is a shiny piece of art, I am sure, in the eyes of a tool and die maker. Designated the "Head Disassembly Instrument," it is used during a hip revision operation, when an impacted steel femoral head must be removed from the prosthetic hip stem without damaging the stem. Any stress put on the stem during this procedure could cause premature failure of the steel hip stem, so it is crucial that the head be removed smoothly and effortlessly. This is made possible by slipping the hip ball inside the instrument's housing, tightening an adjustment nut on its shaft, and then simply squeezing the handle on the other end of the instrument, being careful not to damage the hip stem when removing the steel head. Sound simple enough? Well, as any orthopedic surgeon will tell you, nothing is simple in this business, but the disassembly instrument makes the job a lot smoother than it could be, and, of course, that's good news for the patient.

jaws and the shank. Cement also likes to hide in the tiny crevices of the serrated jaws, of which there are at least three types, on a typical hemostat-like device.

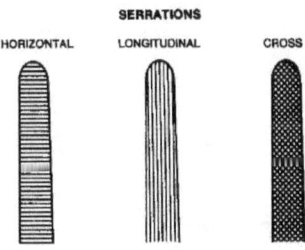

SERRATIONS

HORIZONTAL   LONGITUDINAL   CROSS

Tissue forceps have been known to be major culprits in retaining barely visible shards of bone and tissue in the v-shaped crevice that receives the sharp pointed tip.

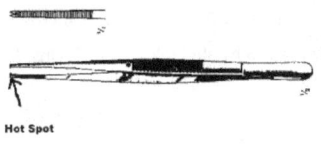

Hot Spot

The Adson Tissue forcep is a special application in its class of instruments, and is used mostly in operations on small bones, such as the bones in the hand, and is also frequently used in vascular and micro- surgery. You may find unwanted tissue lodged in the same manner as in the regular tissue forceps.

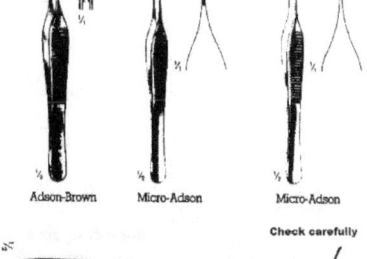

Adson-Brown   Micro-Adson   Micro-Adson

Check carefully

This is a bone currette, used for scraping out tiny chunks of bone. Guess where you will find stubborn fragments of bone or cement?

Here's a closer look at a bone ronguer, this one a Kerrison. These are used in complex operations such as neuro surgery and laminectomies. Sterile Prep initially hand washes these instruments before running them in the ultrasonic machine, which uses ultrasonic vibrations to loosen bioburden from crevices and joints. They are then run through the automatic washer to further reduce the possibility of "hitch-hiking" bone and/or cement.

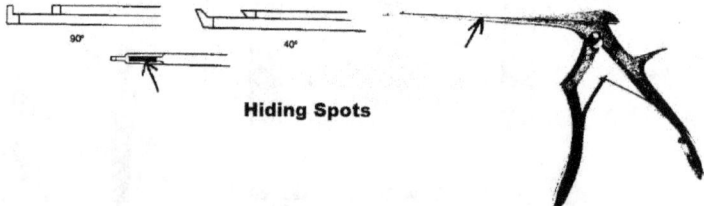

Hiding Spots

On top of the next page, you will see three different types of large bone ronguers, used for such operations as ortho laminectomies, hip surgeries, and other large bones. As I stated in last month's article, it is relatively easy to search out the bone that accumulates inside the jaws of these gouging instruments, but quite another task to remove every minute piece that may be stuck to the hinges of the double-jointed shanks. These are what you might call the "hot spots" on these pliers type ronguers. This is where you would look for any bioburden.

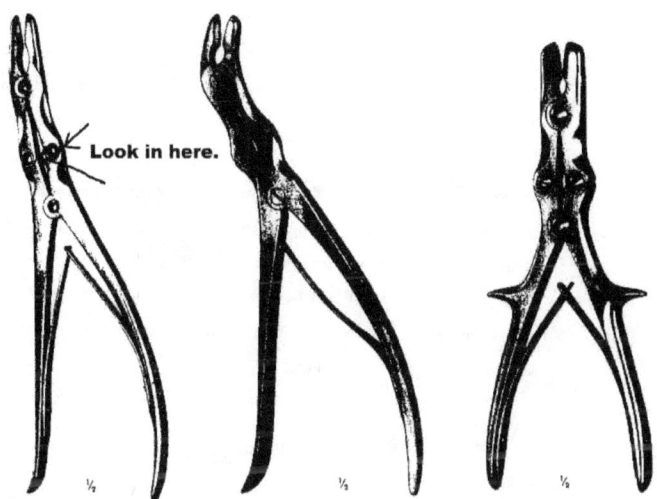

Look in here.

It may come as a surprise to some, but even Mayo-Hegar needle holders are not exempt from retaining bone chips in the tiny cross-hairs of their jaws. These instruments come as a standard item inside the Total Hip Nurses tray, so without a doubt, they are used in large bone cases. Pay close attention to the jaws that have the dished out surfaces.

Look closely

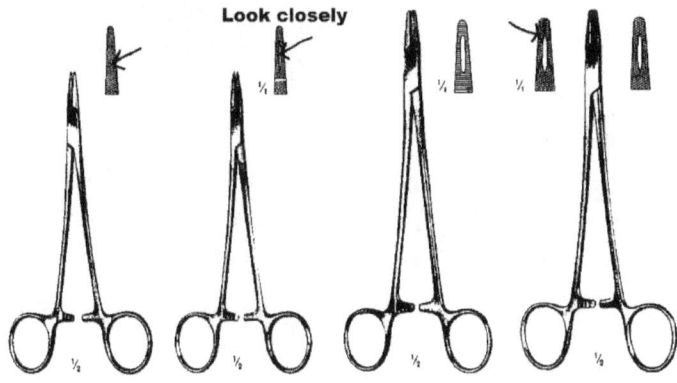

My final study this month is on any bone holding device. Our two most
frequently used bone holders   are Lanes and Lowmanns.
Lanes look like a pair of pliers and can accumulate bone and tissue in
their large serrated jaws. They come in three sizes. Lowmanns look like
a large claw, with a tensioning screw for adjustment. The Lowmann can
also retain bioburden in its jaws, and has the added distinction of being
able to hide bone and tissue between its two joints, so it must be
disassembled before cleaning. Well, that is all for now, so do a fine job
and inspect those instruments!

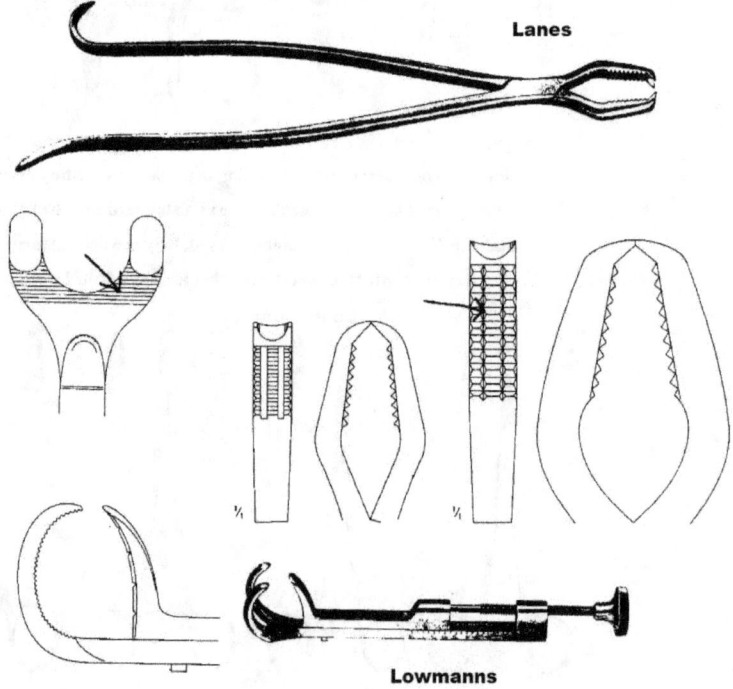

Lanes

Lowmanns

The Art of Sterilization

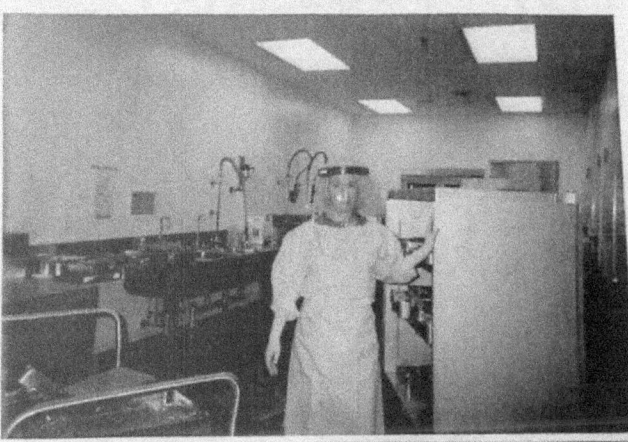

Carts are brought down from the OR and rolled into Decontam, where the soiled instruments are soaked, hand washed, and then placed into a multi-cycle automatic washer, to ensure that every instrument is clean before it arrives in the "clean side" of Sterile Prep. All cannulated instruments are placed into an ultrasonic washer, which removes bioburden through the use of ultrasonic vibration.

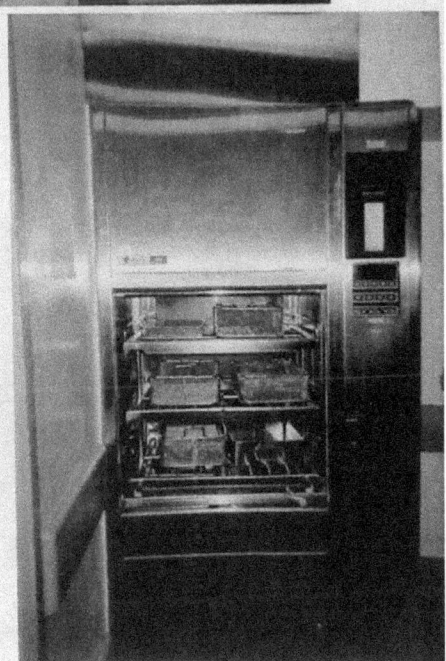

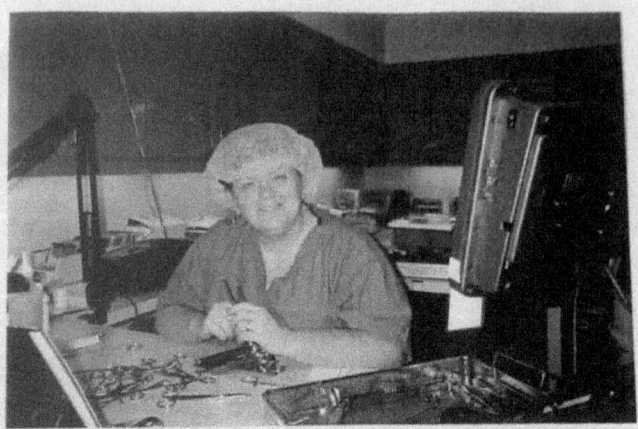

Once the clean instruments are removed from the automatic washers on the sterile side of the department, they are then ready to "assemble." Actually, the term is misleading, as the instruments do not require assembly; they must be sorted out and placed in their proper containers, which could be either a basket (above) or the large modular "toolboxes" that are used in most orthopedic cases (below).

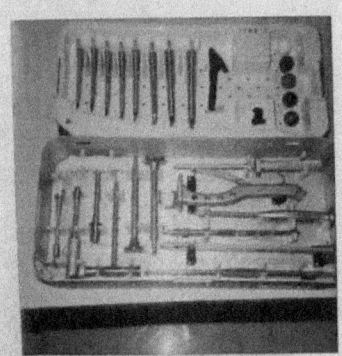

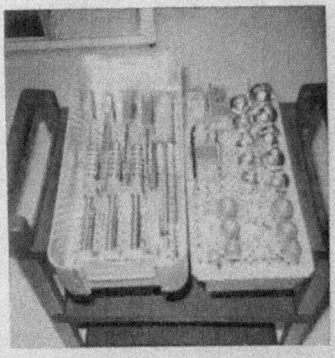

Summit BiPolar
DePuy J+J Hip

The third and final stage in the sterilization process is, you guessed it, the sterilizing stage. About 95% of the instruments that are processed in Sterile Prep can be steam sterilized; The remaining 5% are sterilized in a machine that uses peroxide as a sterilant, usually because these instruments are too delicate to withstand the temperatures of steam sterilization. Instrument trays are either wrapped by hand or placed in metal containers, and wheeled into the autoclave, where they will go through an automatic sterilization process, which takes a total of two hours, from the time the door closes until the trays are cooled and ready for handling. They are then sent back up to the OR. Well, that's it; nothing magic about it, just a lot of work and TLC.

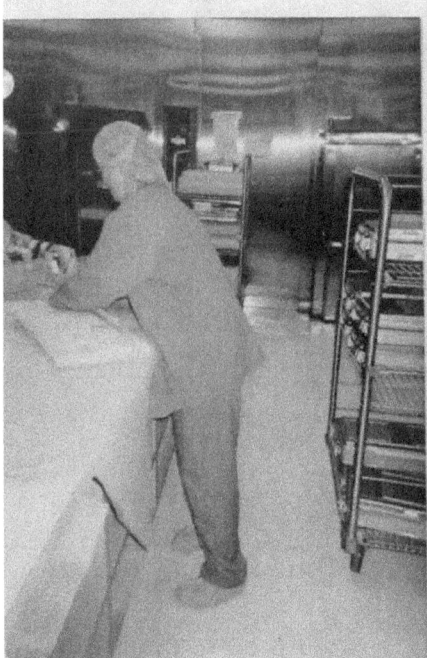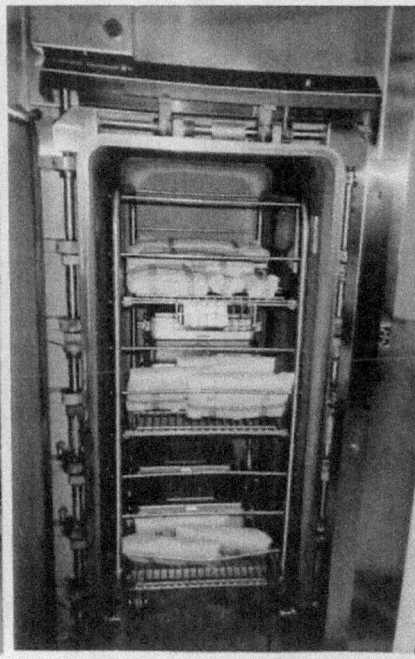

Pictures From the Past

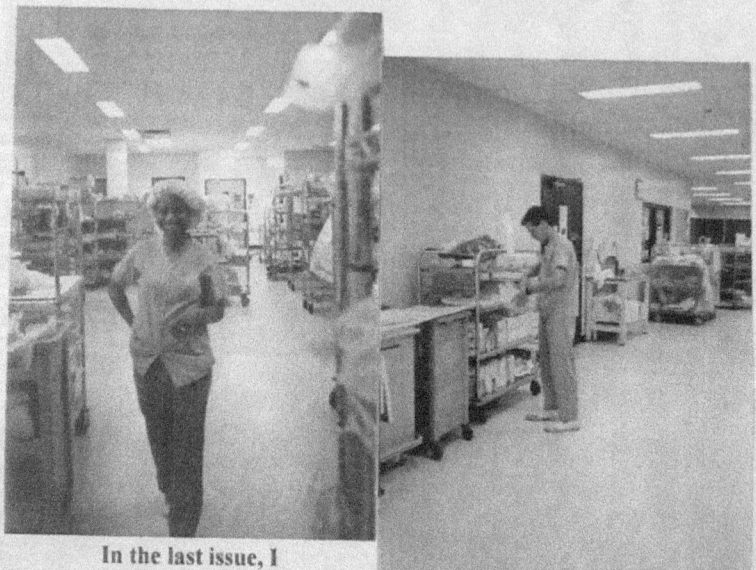

In the last issue, I mentioned that the Sterile Prep Dept. received a facelift a few years ago. Here is former Tech. Fannie standing in front of the vast expanse of the former dept.

Here is a former SPD Tech. looking for supplies in the hallway outside of Decontam that is now dubbed the "corridor of carts." Both these pictures are circa 1988.

Well, friends, gotta go. I hope that you have enjoyed the July issue. It has been a pleasure researching the information for you. See ya.

The Sterile Prep

Times

August 2004

5th Edition

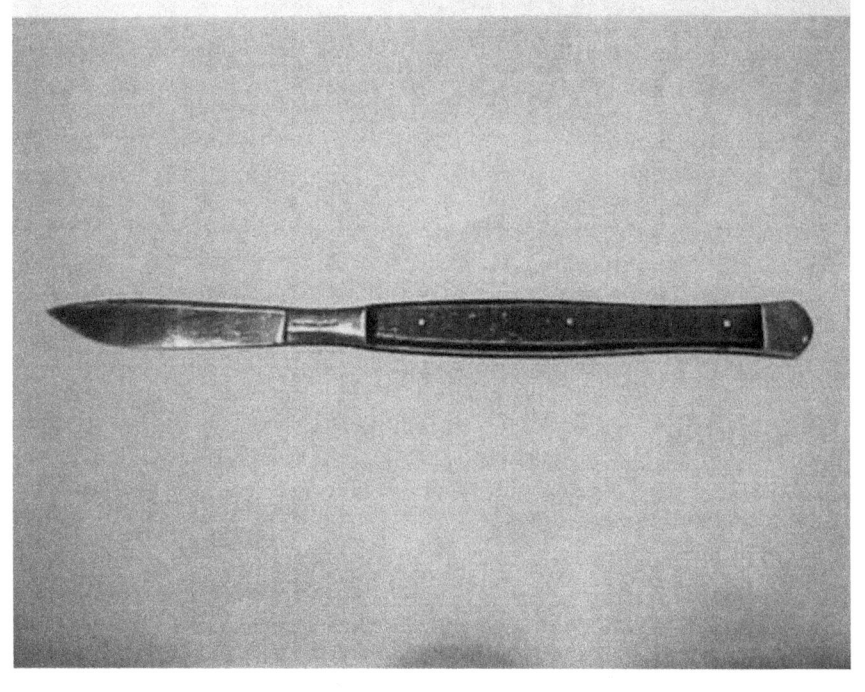

Table of Contents

How Does It Work?

Since this month's Feature Article goes way back in time, when new technologies such as anesthesia and sterilization were first taking root, almost any instrument in use today would contrast sharply with the tools of the trade in the 19th century on back. In fact, about the only instruments still being used in the 21st century that are actual replicas of their 200-year-old counterparts are basic tools such as the saw (for amputation), bone hooks, and chisels. One could argue that the trephine used by a brain surgeon to relieve pressure on a patient's brain has not changed much in the past 200 years or so, which is actually a tribute to the surgical insight of early surgeons.

Occasional similarities aside, the world of medicine in the 21st century is as exciting and innovative as the technology that will someday transport human beings to Mars and beyond. And this month's instrument(s) are true examples of one of the most advanced fields of surgical procedure commonly practiced today: LAPAROSCOPY.

Laparoscopy, although not an entirely new concept, has become increasingly popular as we enter a new era of micro-invasive medicine. The benefits to the patient are significant; very little post-op scar tissue and reduced down time. And the technological breakthroughs just never seem to stop coming. I promise that in an issue of *SPT* in the not-to-distant future, I will do an exclusive Feature Article on laparoscopic surgery. I can feel it in my bones. For this issue though, let's take a look at a couple of examples of state-of-the-art instrumentation, just to whet your appetite.

Here we go. This is the latest in skin staplers, the Tyco TA 60 Auto Suture. This is more or less a universal-type skin stapler. The tissue being sutured is held in place by the clamping device, activated by squeezing the trigger once. Squeeze it a second time and the staple is riveted in place. Single patient use only. Hence, the plastic sealed package.

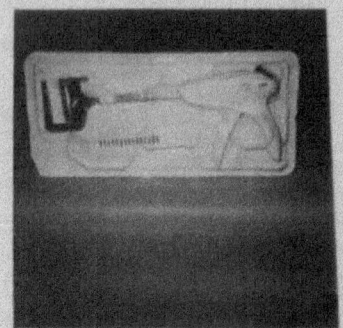

TA 60 Auto Suture

Take a gander at this baby, will ya? Is this hi-tech enough? The Tyco Premium Plus CEEA can be used in surgeries pertaining to the alimentary canal, which is actually a technical term for the entire digestive tract. The long, slender, curved body of the device is actually inserted in the digestive tube, and staples are fired away in sections that no other stapler could possibly reach. Can you say, "Wow!"

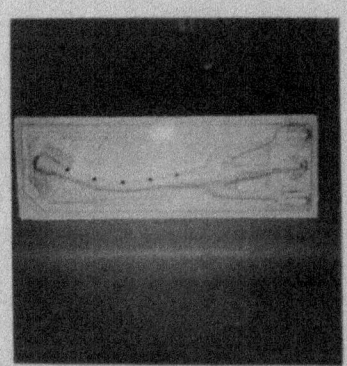

Premium Plus CEEA
Auto Suture

In The Field

This month's Feature Article by Rick Hughes

Welcome to this month's Feature column. I hope you have enjoyed reading this issue of *SPT* thus far. This is the section that was described in the Introduction as "breaking the mold." During the past month, since the completion of the July issue, I have been researching the history of field sterilization, its applications, and the different methods of providing sterile instruments to surgeons in the field. As I became immersed in the study of the different facets of the delivery of medical care during the various wars, conflicts, and battles, I was reminded of all the sacrifices and tremendous PAIN that our forefathers experienced in service to their country. And so I dedicate this column to all the men and women who have served their country, all over the world, and especially here in the U.S., defending freedom and our way of life. Somehow you all make the rest of us feel like mere mortals, and we hope that the country that you have helped so much to shape will always be worthy of the sacrifices that have been made to preserve it. The fact that you did it all in the name of FREEDOM moves us. And we thank you.

Another fact that hit home while I was studying medicine in the field is the importance of sterilization. You know, as Americans in the 21st century, we are pretty jaded. We've seen it all, and not only that, but we have been seeing it for years now. Sterilized instruments in the surgical field is so taken for granted, so expected, that it is hard to envision a time or a place where this was, and in some cases IS, not always the case.

When the early European settlers came over to the New World, they found a relatively primitive culture, the North American Indian. These Native Americans were bound by traditions that were hundreds, sometimes thousands of years old. Yet, although it is a popular belief that their only medicine consisted of the sprinkling of "magic dust" or the drinking of potions, in fact the Indians were pretty crafty when it came to healing the sick and wounded. Contrary to what one might think, tribal medicine men did perform surgeries, and the mortality rates were likely no worse (if not more favorable) than those of the field docs during the Civil War, whose methods of sterilization were questionable, at best. Because I have no statistics on those early Native American patients, it would be difficult to say just how successful the medicine men were at treating serious wounds. Yet, we know that they always used natural ingredients in their surgeries, as in all their other facets of life, so we can surmise that they likely boiled their primitive instruments before using them. It is clear from the studies of North American tribal medicine that the Indians did in fact understand the necessity of aseptic techniques in surgery. Of course, when the settlers came over from Europe, they found the Indian ways too primitive for their liking, and so they spread the word that the medicine men were no more than "witch doctors", their cures no more than hoaxes.

Yet, those early American doctors were practicing medicine that was scarcely more sterile and safe than the Native medicine men's craft. It was not until Joseph Lister began studying asepsis in surgery, back in 1865 that the medical community was made aware of the importance of sterility in surgery. Later, in 1878, German Robert Koch had discovered a method of steam sterilizing instruments and dressings. These discoveries had been long overdue. You see, the American Civil War, fought between 1861 and 1865, by far the bloodiest and costliest battle ever fought on American soil, was a surgeon's nightmare. Field doctors operated on wooden tables, either out in the open or under the slight protection of makeshift tents. The most common form of anesthetic was a bottle of whiskey, which the patient was given right before the operation. The most common type of operation was, by far, amputation. Sterility of surgical instruments and bandages did not exist. The mortality rate was through the roof. Of the soldiers who had to have amputations at the hip joint, less than 20% survived. Even a BKA rendered about a 50/50 survival rate. These were men who might have made it through the battle, had the field surgeon been able to use sterile instruments on his patients, instead of merely wiping off the blood between operations. This is just one of the countless tragic footnotes from the Civil War that hopefully have served to teach us the WRONG way to do things.

In the following pages, for your review, I have included some notable pictures from the Civil War era, downloaded from various websites.

The Field Surgeon and His Instruments
During The Civil War

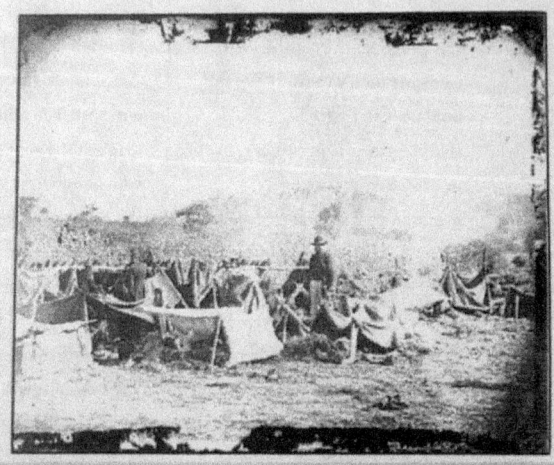

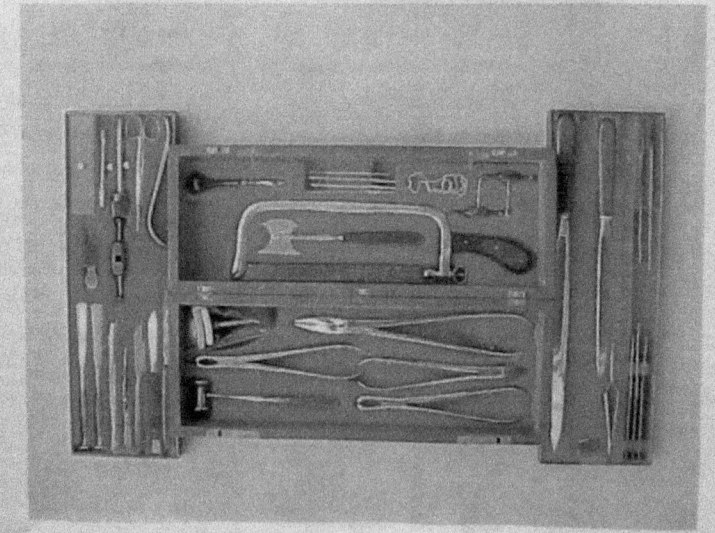

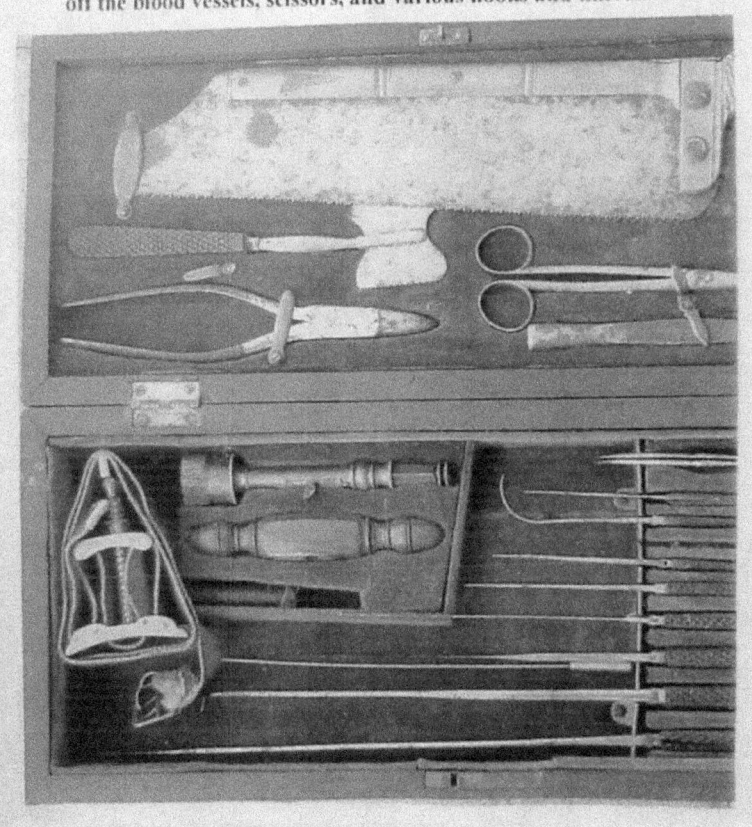

Here you see a typical field doctor's instrument case, representative of the most common tools used in field surgery. As indicated earlier, the saw was the most popular instrument used in the field during the Civil War. Also visible are a trephine, to relieve pressure on the brain, a tourniquet to close off the blood vessels, scissors, and various hooks and knives.

By the time World War I began, aseptic surgery had become common practice. As a result, the majority of GI's who were treated for wounds received on the battlefield survived and lived to fight another day. That does not make war any safer than it used to be, but a soldier's chances of surviving a bullet wound to the leg are MUCH better than they were in the 19th century, before the practice of sterilization of instruments became commonplace. Still, the cold realities of wartime surgery hit hard, and it is hard for some to even imagine operating or being operated on under a tent, in a war zone. Here are some pictures of a simulated MASH unit, where modern-day civilians re-create the actions of military medical personnel in emergency situations, using authentic props. Notice the Army issue sterilzer.

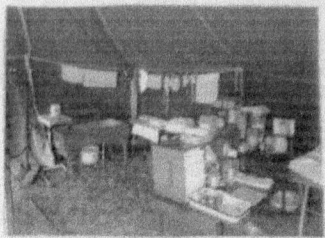

Steam Sterilizer

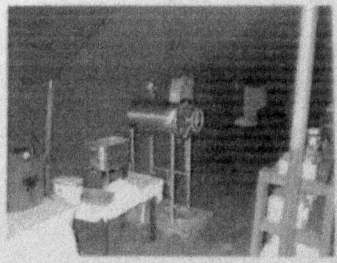

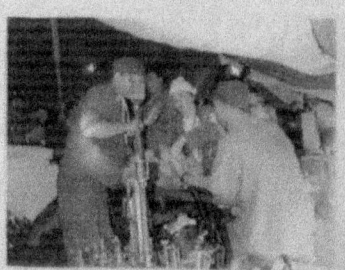

Because of the valiant and courageous work of the medics who have treated the wounded and saved lives during all of the various wars, other heroic feats in the annals of field medicine are often overlooked. Case in point: think of all the men and women who volunteer to treat the sick and the wounded in Third World countries that lack their own medical facilities. The conditions under which these medical miracle workers perform should automatically reserve for them a beach condo in Heaven. Left to their own devices, the native people of these impoverished places would surely die from untreated diseases. But real people with BIG hearts reach deep within themselves, realize that they can save some lives, and do what they feel is necessary. And in this writer's mind, these lifesavers are every bit as brave and heroic as any soldier who has ever signed up for duty overseas. Places such as Kenya, Zimbabwe, Tanzania, and other areas of destitution, far out of sight, and also out of most of our thoughts, often become personal feats of triumph to medical personnel who decide on making it their personal goal to rid an entire community of disease. Hats off to you all!

In keeping with our theme of field sterilization, I have included, along with a couple of pictures of an obviously poverty-stricken hospital in Tanzania, a picture of a surgeon taking a break between operations in Kenya. Notice the pressure cooker behind him, used for the sterilization of instruments. This method, although somewhat archaic, is actually 100% effective, and has proven a valuable tool in Third World countries.

This is the Kilindoni Hospital, located on Mafia Island, Tanzania, in southeastern Africa. What appears to be an abandoned shack is actually a sanctuary for the sick.

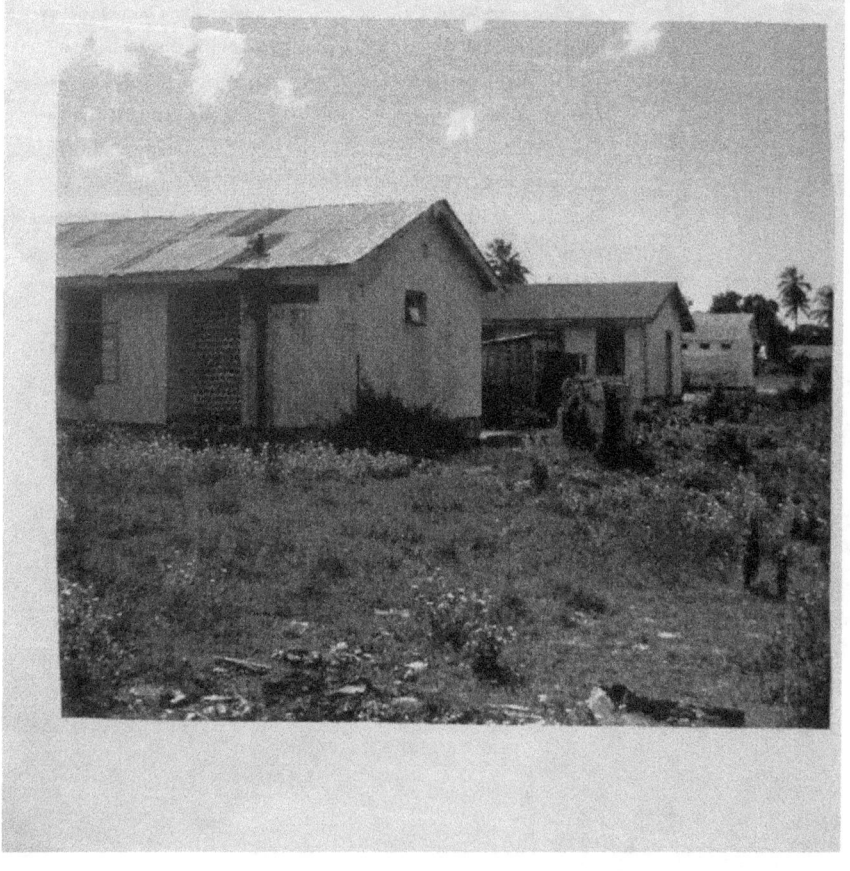

Here we have a clinic examination room inside the Kilindoni Hospital ward in Tanzania. Although the surroundings look "second-rate", all the equipment appears to be clean. Under the circumstances, the surgery performed here, assuming the surgeons are proficient, should be quite safe. Ultimately, the degree of sterility is the key to a safe operation. Remember, only 100% is safe.

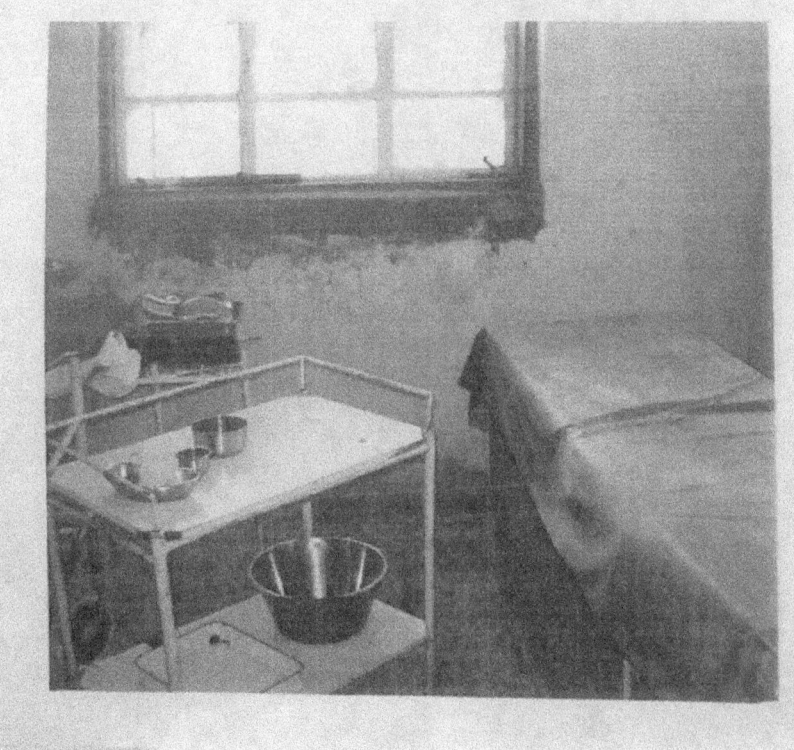

And here is the good doctor, smiling between cases, with the aforementioned pressure cooker/sterilizer in the background. What keeps this guy smiling? Something tells me it is not his salary.

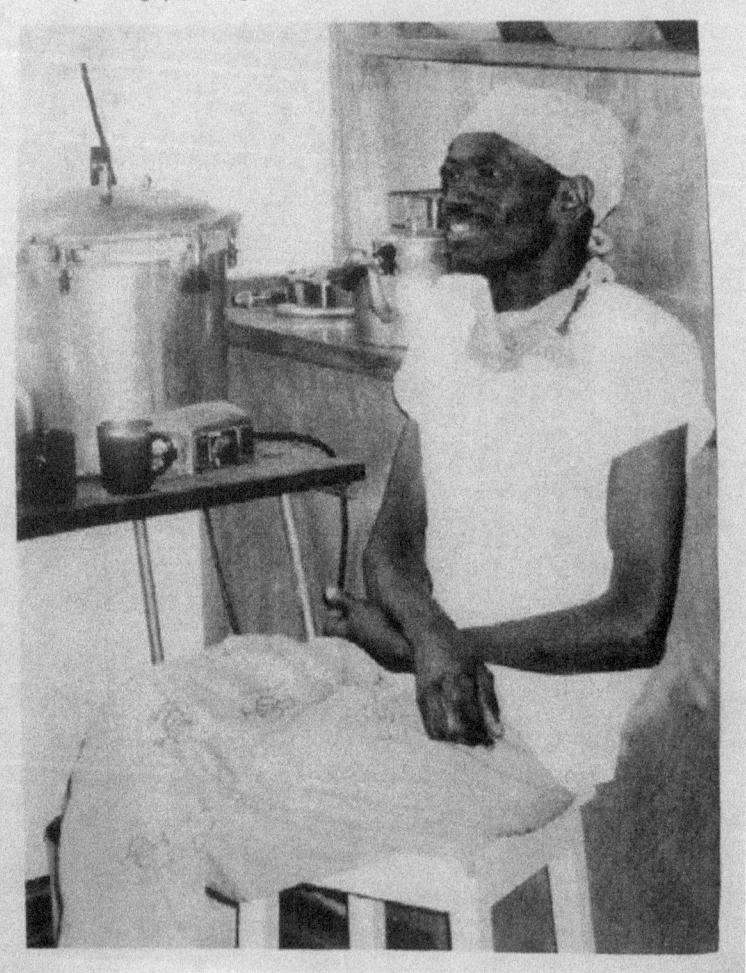

So there you have it; the results of my research of field sterilization, from before its widespread use after the Civil War, to the present. The basic design, as you have seen through the use of the pictures, has not changed much, since the principle is still the same. All that is required is to kill ALL the bacteria AND the spores. And the uses are endless; the sterilization of hemostats to save a baby's life in Mozambique; or the removal of a bullet in war-torn Iraq. In other words, sterile instruments are critical, and field sterilization is the key to operating in far-off lands.

And what about the future of field sterilization? Is the technology changing? Well, there's a silly question. As we have seen, medical technology is constantly on the move. Check out this Infrared Sterilizer manufactured by LEEDS. Built about the size of an average portable unit, Model 1 (its designation) operates without steam or chemicals, has no toxic emissions, and is self-cleaning. According to its literature, the LEEDS Model 1 "uses infrared technology to rapidly sterilize medical instruments without corrosion damage..." There is your future.

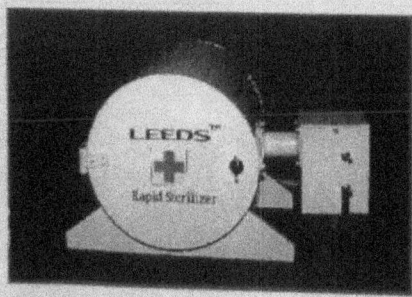
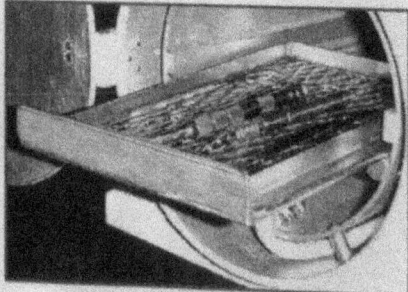

Well, what do you know? Another issue of *SPT* is behind us. Once again, I have really enjoyed gathering all the information necessary to bring you, the reader, an interesting yet informative look into our world of sterilization and instrumentation. And while you are reading this issue with captivating pleasure, rest assured that this writer is concocting something even more novel and innovative for the next issue, the 6th Edition. Even though the September issue is merely in its dreamlike form at this time, let me give you some ideas I have been throwing around. Let's see, there are, of course, the usual forums, OR Links, How Does It Work? , etc. .... For next month, I am currently looking into writing an article about robotics, maybe a study of sterile processing departments on hospital ships, and an interview with one of Sterile Prep's youngest and brightest stars. Until then, I sincerely hope you have enjoyed the August issue, and to all of you out there who make this hospital a brighter place to work I say,

"Keep Rollin'."

The Sterile Prep Times

September 2004

6th Edition

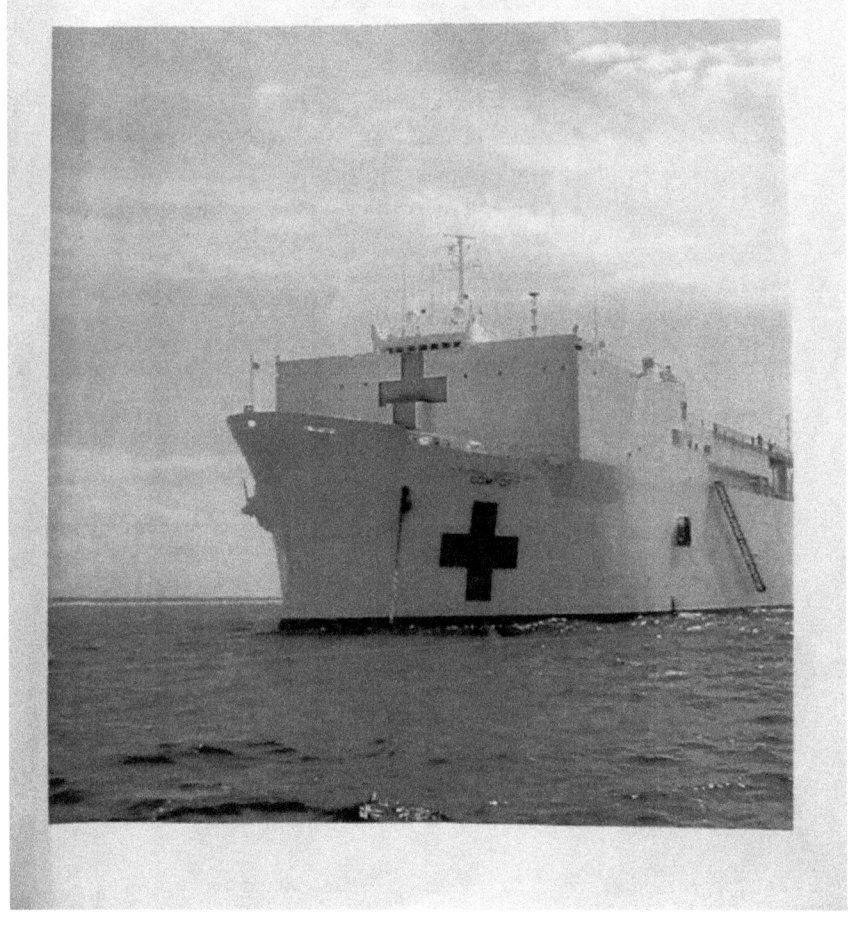

Table of Contents

The Sterile Prep Times

6th Edition   September 2004

Hello again. Here we are, heading into the Fall already. Not that it will mean a change in the weather, mind you, just that summer is almost over. And we all know what that means; SEASON. More people, more traffic, more stress, more... well, you get the idea. However, it also means more business to the entrepreneurs among us. To those of us in Surgical Services, it means only one thing: more surgeries; lots more. I wish I could say something here to help you all get through the coming busy season with less stress and anxiety and, most of all, more energy. Unfortunately, I am not Spiderman. I will, however, recommend watching the TV show "Scrubs." I've only seen it a couple of times (I don't watch much TV), and it really takes your mind off of the seriousness of our business, if only for a half-hour. So, watch the show once a week, take the dog for a walk every now and then, spend a couple of hours just sitting by the ocean watching the waves (there ARE waves in the Fall), and then take a deep breath before work each day, and you should be alright. Works for me.

Hey, did you all enjoy last month's *Times* ? I think it was my favorite, so far, although I really think that this issue kicks butt, too. This could be the last of my lengthy newsletters for awhile (I will explain later), so let's hope that it is received really well this month. There is some really cool stuff in this issue, I've done all my homework, so find yourself a nice cozy spot to take a ten-minute break, and let's get started.....

How Does It Work?

Medical Robotics

A writer never knows who will be reading his work: Young or old; male or female; college student or dedicated nine-to-fiver. However, in a closed environment such as the hospital setting, a good percentage of the readership is going to be medically oriented. The reason I am throwing this statistic at you is pure and simple. There are certain subjects that interest this author, being medically oriented myself, and I cannot help but wonder if there are more of you out there who also find these things fascinating. There have been at least a couple of instances in the latest issues of *The Times* where the subject matter seemed to have little to do with this hospital, and I admit that. Yet, comparing the quality of care received in two different centuries, or two different countries in the *same* century, is information that we can use; it is certainly interesting enough to merit an article in the Special Feature section of this newsletter. And, of course, I hope that you will agree.

This month, I want you to take a look at one of the directions that medicine is definitely going, and you can decide for yourself whether or not the future is bright in our field. The subject is *medical robotics,* and it has been in the hearts and minds of scientists around the world for quite awhile now. As we keep pressing ahead in our computerized world, is it possible, or even *practical,* that someday robots will be performing such complex and delicate operations as neuro and vascular surgery?

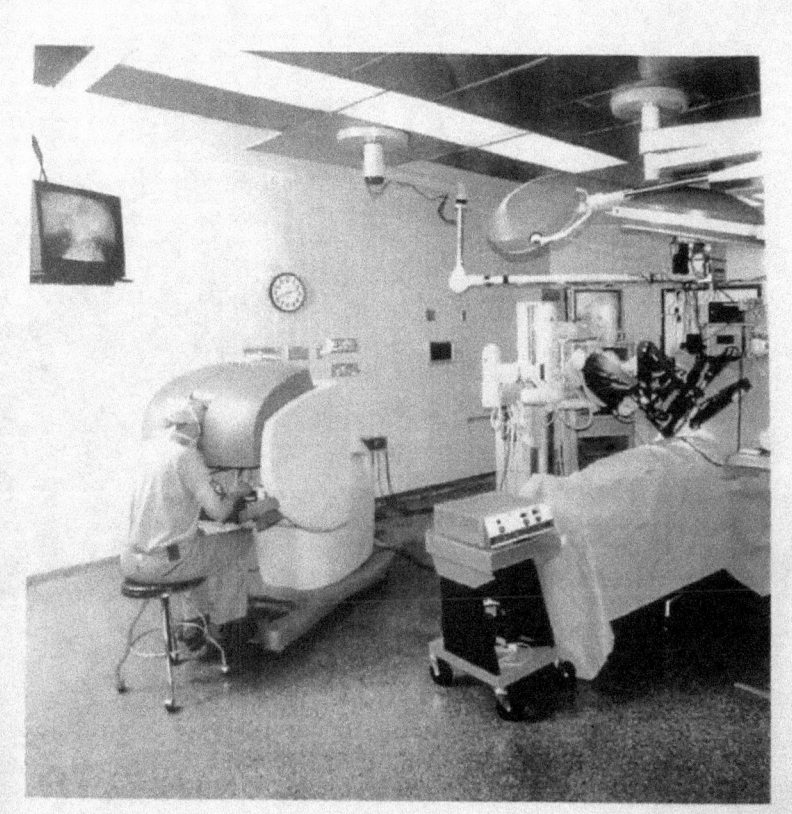

This is the Da Vinci System. The surgeon sits at a console in the same room as the patient, currently required by the FDA, and operates hand controls and foot pedals that manipulate the robot arms.

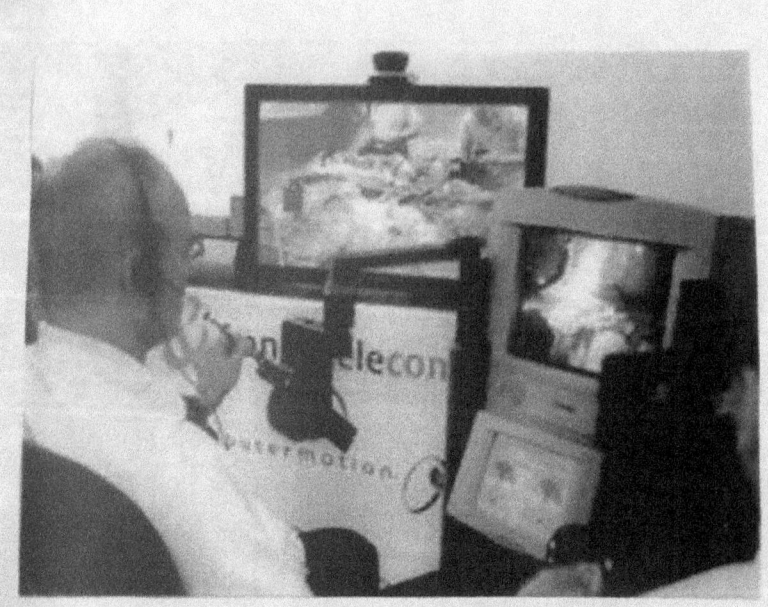

Here, a doctor performs what is known as "remote control robotic surgery" on a patient who is thousands of miles away. This type of operation is said to be opening doors for patients that need a certain doctor or specialist who may be living and working on the other side of the globe. Soldiers on the battlefield are also potential beneficiaries of this system, where the surgeon can manipulate robot arms by voice commands and hand controls, as well, without leaving his monitor.

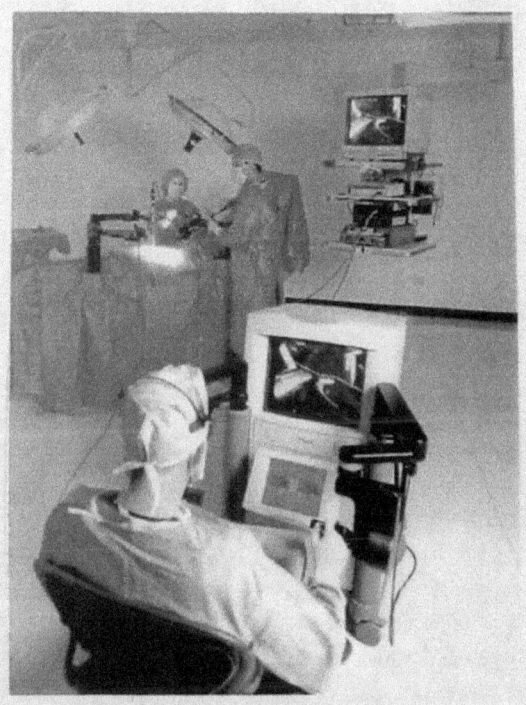

In this photo, the surgeon operates the robotic arms with voice commands generated through a headset. He can also use hand and finger-operated controls, as the task dictates. This type of robotic arm is becoming more common, and even small community-based hospitals such as IRMH utilize some type of robotics. In certain surgeries where a machine-like grip is needed, whether to manipulate a retractor, for example, or to hold a camera steady, robots give the surgeon a hand.

Special Feature:
Hospital Ships

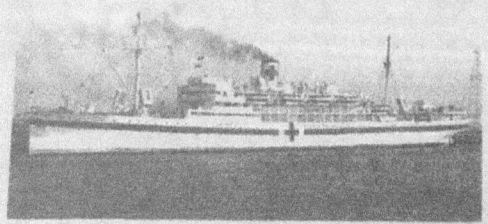

Many of the hospital ships used in World War II were converted from troop transports, such as the USAHS Thistle, shown in the picture above. Today, the United States Navy commissions two large vessels for the medical treatment of casualties during overseas operations: the USNS Comfort, shown at right, and the USNS Mercy, both converted supertankers. As you can see, the Comfort is equipped with a helo pad, to receive both supplies and medevac patients.

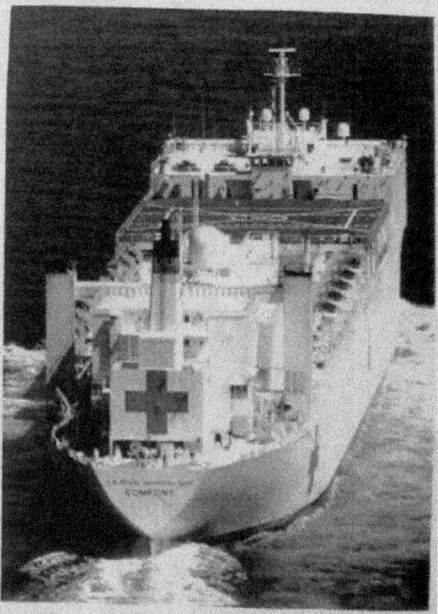

We live in an ever-changing society, one that encourages, among other objectives, progress, technology, and comfort. With each passing generation, we strive to overcome the limits of the previous one, always hoping for breakthroughs in the important issues of medicine, energy, food, and peace among nations. In essence, we take pride in making this world a better place to live, for the present and future generations of its inhabitants. All things considered, the free world has succeeded in improving almost every aspect of the human condition, and the United States has been instrumental in making it happen. The yearning for peace and prosperity has transported us from a rural, somewhat backward society of the 17th and 18th centuries, to the computer-literate culture that we enjoy today.

Of course, for our purposes, we are most interested in the extensive developments in medicine over the years. Last month, I intended to illustrate the improvements in field medicine, from the Civil War era to the present. In doing so, one cannot help but notice how much we now take health care for granted, as long as we are at home, in the U.S. For sure, the greatest concern nowadays about medical needs and emergencies is how one can afford it, without good insurance. Otherwise, our confidence in the abilities of the physicians to "fix" whatever is wrong with us is such that a patient can rightly expect to survive an operation that, until recently (meaning over the past ten or fifteen years), could have proven extremely dangerous. We owe a great deal to the pioneers of medicine.

Also evident in last month's article was how important it has always been to be able to mobilize medicine, especially during times of war. Medics, or corpsmen, have been as much a part of the infantry as the soldiers on the front line, always there when called upon, always risking their lives to save others. With little more than a briefcase full of instruments, they have been asked to perform everything from a broken arm to an open chest wound and worse. And then there were the MASH personnel; the nurses, surgeons, and corpsmen who operated out of a makeshift hospital, just beyond the front lines. Those tents, with the huge red crosses emblazoned on their canopies, were shelters in the storm, a sight for sore eyes, to a wounded and tired GI.

Some battlegrounds, however, did not afford the "luxury" of MASH units or anything else resembling a hospital on dry land. Vietnam for example, was characterized by its jungle warfare and Riverine operations, which consisted of small crafts patrolling up and down the meandering waterways of the Mekong River. Soldiers wounded during these operations were either airlifted to a medical facility, whenever possible, or transported to a medical aid boat, which always accompanied the troop-carrying boats in their riverine operations. These medical aid boats carried one medical Corps officer and seven medics, as well as a radio operator. They had at their disposal a basic field medical and surgical set, and a refrigerator full of whole blood. Night operations required a helicopter pilot of great skill to land on the boat's small deck.

Contrast the description of the medical aid boats in Vietnam with those of the two enormous hospital ships utilized by the United States Navy today, and you will see that there is really no comparison. As seen in the photo on the above right, there was very little room with which to work in the Mekong Delta, in 1966.

In the photo on the right, below, American soldiers in Vietnam had to work in cramped conditions whenever a comrade was transported from the helicopter to the landing deck, and then to the cargo deck for medical treatment. Compare this with the size of the USNHS Comfort's deck, as shown in this article's title page, and you get a good idea of the difference in these two vessels. Like apples and oranges.

(Thanks to the Mobile Riverine Force Association for the info. Photos courtesy of Albert Moore, President, MRFA.)

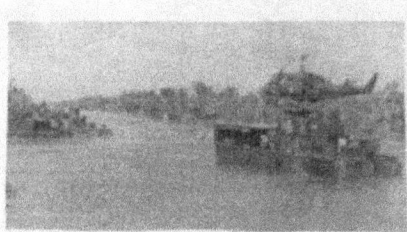

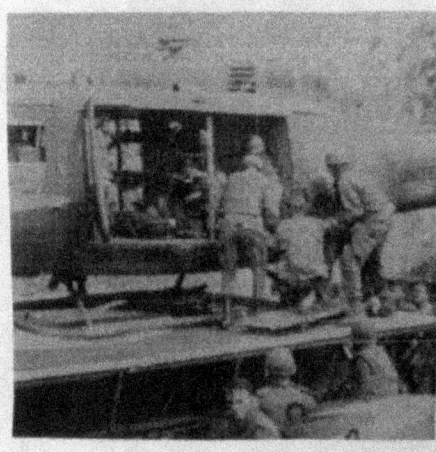

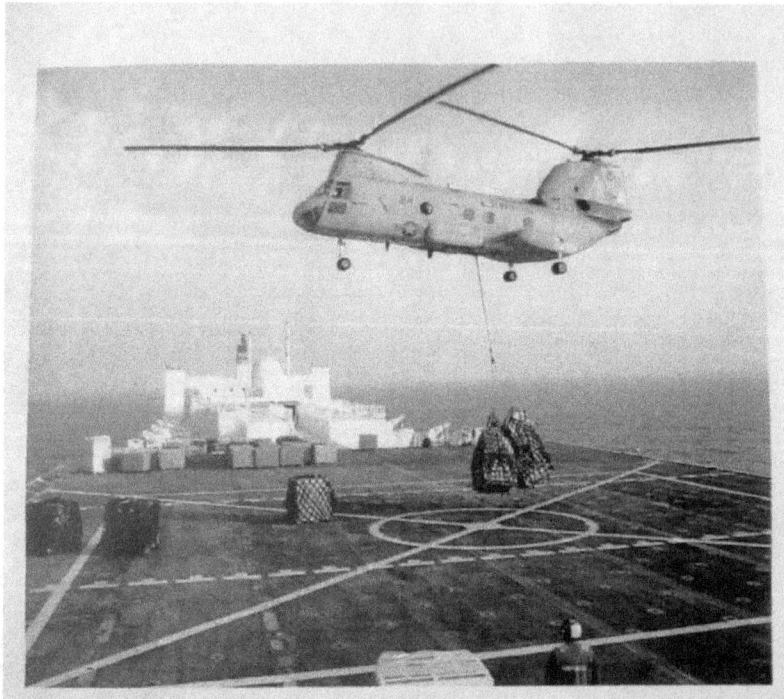

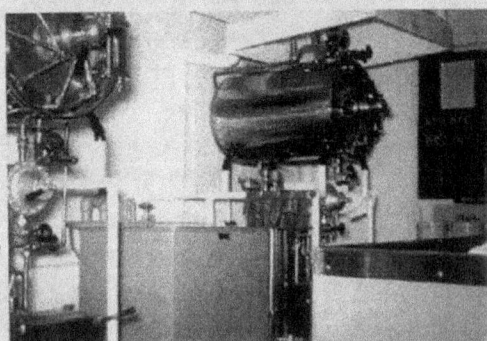

(Above): A USN transport chopper drops off supplies on the Comfort's deck. (Right): Steam sterilizers on board the Army Hospital Ship Thistle, circa 1944.

From these stark comparisons, one might judge prematurely that working on a hospital ship more closely resembles being employed in a "regular" hospital than it does a MASH unit or other makeshift medical facility. And, in at least one sense, that being the comfort factor, they would be right. However, a closer look at history shows that hospital ships have the dubious reputation of being a favorite target of the enemy, while in international waters. Ironic and cruel as it seems, ships with big red crosses emblazoned across their bows have been sunk with reckless abandon, since their institution during the first World War. It is a bleak statement on human nature that any vessel loaded down with sick people would be engaged in battle, especially when you consider that the hospital ships, under the Geneva Convention, have never been allowed to possess weaponry, rendering them completely defenseless. Tragically, many lives have been lost aboard hospital ships, both patients and crews.

Although modern warfare is no safer than ancient warfare (the object is still to kill or maim people), somehow I just can't imagine any of our present-day enemies being able to attack either of the US Navy's hospital ships, the Mercy or the Comfort. After 9/11, you have to believe that they have the full protection of the US military's firepower. Yet, we know, too, that the terrorists are capable of merciless mass destruction, and are willing to risk anything to destroy anything American. In any case, the crews of these two vessels (about 1200 strong each), like the rest of our soldiers abroad, deserve our prayers.

10 WORKING WITH GOD

Some would say that a hospital is a hospital is a hospital. Others might argue that besides the size of a facility and its various specialties, the most distinguishing feature is whether it is a religious hospital, a non-denominational, profit, not-for-profit, or government run (V.A.) hospital. Before you start preparing for a no-holds-barred scientific comparison between every type of hospital that exists today in the United States, set your brain back on **CASUAL** mode. We're not going to compare any of them. We're not even going to cover all of them. The main idea of this chapter is to let you the reader know how God and prayer can improve your work experience.

If you should read or have already read my book

(Bless you) **Mowing at the Master's Level**, you will see how one can embrace a typically thankless job like the lawn business. If you haven't read it yet I will only tell you that I wrote an entire book, albeit a rather short one, on the subject of mowing grass. It isn't instructional, nor does it discuss the technical aspects of mower repair or running a business. It is simply about the joys of mowing for the Lord. It is possible to find joy in any occupation, whether it is one we have always wanted to do or one that we feel stuck in. That last statement might have some readers shaking their heads. How is it possible to find joy in work that drains every ounce of energy out of your body each day? How about a job that you no longer find interesting or challenging because you have been doing it for ten years or more and it has never changed? Have you thought about what would happen if you are making good money in sterile processing ten years from now but the job is driving you nuts? It can happen and in fact it does happen to a lot of good workers. There are several scenarios that could actually make one feel stuck in his or her job as a sterile processing technician with nowhere to go but down. It's not the worst place to be but it sure does make it hard to go to work every day. It's important to choose your career wisely because you never know how far you can take it. It's like the old saying: Be careful what you wish for. In your early days as a new technician you might hope beyond hope that someday you will actually make good money doing your job. Well guess what? It's like I stated earlier in the book, some hospitals are paying pretty decent wages these days for sterile processing techs; WAY more than we ever dreamed of back in the 1990's in our small town. The job is a lot more technical nowadays with all the fancy instruments and computerized equipment but it is still basically the same job. An old tech can learn a few new tricks and still compete with all the new tech-savvy employees coming out of high school or traveling from around the country. Never worked with travelers before? You will. Sterile processing is becoming more and more *visible* in the hospital with each passing year. As it becomes more popular there will be more skilled workers in the trade whose desire it is to travel around the country, or even the world, working as an SPT.

Whatever career you choose, whether you feel yourself drawn to sterile processing or something totally different, the key to being successful or having longevity in your job is to embrace it. Even if you are not sure if it is your calling, any work you do that involves healing the sick is Jesus' work, so embrace it. If there is something better for you down the road God will open your eyes to it. Have faith.

In my case God never fully opened the door to any other career after I started working in sterile processing, and whenever He did I didn't have the faith it took to carry me through. As a result I never really embraced my job in Central until I was 60 years old. This is neither a lie nor a stretching of the truth. As illustrated in an earlier chapter, I began my career in the hospital hoping to get into the Radiography program. God granted me that opportunity but for some reason I lost the desire to follow that dream through to its fruition. Another decade passed by mowing grass and working in sterile processing, until the opportunity arose once again to go back to college. This time I studied Sociology and ended up receiving my Bachelors degree in Psychology even though I wasn't sure what to do with it. As more time went by I began praying harder that God would show me what direction to go. When I received the call from Orlando, of course my wife and I both thought that was the answer to our prayers. As it turned out, the educator job was just another stepping stone in the quest to find my true calling. Finally, at the age of 60 and with almost 30 years of Central Service under my belt, I came to realize that God had wanted me to be a sterile processing technician all along. I know it sounds crazy but if you had lived in my shoes and had exhausted just about every other possible option for a career by trial and error, you might have come to the same conclusion. I could finish out this chapter or maybe even write a whole book on the details of how I deciphered God's message that He always wanted me to be an SPT, but I don't think that would further anyone's cause really, so you'll just have to take my word for it. Believe me, after thirty years of washing and sterilizing instruments, I wouldn't still be doing this if I didn't think God was calling me to do it. The moral of this story is: While you are waiting for a prayer to be answered, one that you may have been praying for weeks, months, or even years; take a step back and make sure it hasn't been answered already. As it has been said, the Lord works in mysterious ways. That old saying is believed to have been derived from scripture, although it is a rough translation at best. From the book of Isaiah 55:8-9,

"For my thoughts are not your thoughts,

neither are your ways my ways,"

declares the Lord.

"As the heavens are higher than the earth,

so are my ways higher than your ways

and my thoughts than your thoughts."

Another good illustration of this scripture is the story of how I managed to overcome one of the worst broken hearts I ever had to suffer through. I had been in a relationship with a particular young woman for a couple of years. There may have been times when our feelings for each other were mutual, especially at the beginning, but for the most part I was in love and she seemed just 'okay' with that. Not only was it mostly a one-way relationship but she liked to play games too. I was working two full-time jobs so spare time was very rare and precious to me, and I wanted to spend it all with her. Yet she repeatedly stood me up on dates. It was all one way but I didn't see it. I just knew that whenever we were together I was happy. It was a hurtful relationship and I constantly sought the advice of my sister, who always said I was too good for this woman; that I should leave her and find a girl who really loved and cared about me. Yet I wanted her. So I prayed; kneeling at the foot of my bed and praying to God that she would want me just as badly as I wanted her. But it never happened. She continued to break my heart almost every week, until one lonely night I had hurt enough. I kneeled at the foot of my bed at about 11:30pm, my usual time to hit the hay after a long 16-hour day of work. And I prayed to God to take away my pain. He's very good at that you know. I prayed that we would *both have the same feelings for each other*. And you know what? That one worked. The next day I felt the miracle of God working in my soul to make everything right again. He took the pain from my heart, and as for the desire for that woman it was as if *it never existed!* From that moment on whenever we met she was just like a friend to me, a mere acquaintance; no more broken promises, no more broken heart, and best of all no more one-way relationship. It was a miracle. God had not answered my previous prayers because I had been praying for the wrong thing; I had been praying for someone else's feelings to change. In essence, unbeknownst to me I had been praying for that young woman to change her whole life around *for me*. She had three children and a previous broken marriage and for all I know more problems than I could ever imagine. Yet I wanted her to think about me all the time just as I thought about her. In other words I had been praying to God to let me be selfish and also to make her be selfish as well. And God was simply saying "No." He had better plans for both of us.

The young woman who had been the object of my desire for those two emotionally painful years eventually got remarried and moved out of state. She once again lives close to the mountains, a dream she had harbored for many years. I am happy for her. As for me I have been married for almost fifteen years as of this writing, to a woman who really loves and cares about me, a dream I had harbored for many years before I met her. We share a beautiful home and the love of all our kids, grandkids, and our dog. Our relationship is based on God's love and His plan for us together as a couple. We are bonded together in His spirit. We don't always see eye to eye. In fact that is an understatement. My wife is a ten year cancer survivor with physical limitations that keep her from enjoying a lot of the activities we used to do together such as cycling, one of my favorite hobbies. Somewhere along the way her equilibrium has been affected, probably from the chemo treatments that are the bane of almost every patient diagnosed with cancer. But after almost fifteen years of marriage I've learned that it's not all about enjoying sports activities together. Sure, couples who play sports together have something special that should not be taken for granted. But to me marriage is mostly about being able to share God's love with someone the way He wants us to share it. It's about realizing that no man or woman is perfect, no relationship is perfect, and our lives here on Earth are not perfect. And God knows we are not perfect because He created us. Only through our faith and love for Jesus Christ can we ever be perfect in God's eyes because He loves His son so much. That is the best we can do while we are here and that is how my wife and I have chosen to live out our lives together.

Nice stories and I am blessed to call them my own,

but to be true to this chapter's title I must tell you what working with God means to me. I remember working in a tiny sterile processing department when I lived on Florida's east coast. It was so tiny they only had one full-time employee running the whole show. The OR manager hired me part-time to give her some much needed help on the busiest days of the week. She was the nicest lady I had ever worked with and of course a hard worker as well. She never boasted, never complained, never imposed on me to do her work for her, and was always grateful for the help that I did give her. In other words this sweet middle-aged Filipino lady had all the good qualities of a Christian. Yet we never discussed religion. I only helped out at that little hospital for one summer; had I worked there longer perhaps we would have gotten into discussions about God and Jesus. As it was I only assumed she was a believer.

You can always "feel" God at work in a hospital. There is a spirit, The Holy Spirit that holds the entire building in the palm of its hands so to speak, and gives off a positive energy that can turn the worst nightmare of a workday into a blessing. Only God and His angels can do this. And if you don't have either one in your life I hope that one day you will; because even if you don't think you have Him *He has you*, my friend. And like your best friend holding onto the rope on the other end so you don't fall into the pit, He won't let go unless you deny Him. Like your best friend He will not stick around if you shun Him and He will not force Himself upon you. But whenever you ask for Him, God is there.

I have worked in hospitals where our machines would break down more than they were up and running. I remember one week when the instrument washers stopped working on Wednesday and didn't get fixed until Friday. That's almost three days of backed up case carts full of instruments waiting to go into the washers. How could a hospital that performed thirty to thirty-five surgeries per day operate under such conditions? I really can't answer that. All I know is my supervisor was a good Christian woman, a little eccentric and over-zealous at times but good nonetheless, and she never once gave up on God's ability to get us through any kind of day the OR threw at us. Her strength and faith in God made me a believer in her and strengthened my relationship with God and Jesus. One strong Christian really can make a difference.

One final thought before signing off. One of the most useful lessons I have learned is the "portability" of working with God. When you purchase life insurance from your employer one of the things hoped for is that you can take it with you when you leave that particular employer. If not, all the money that went into the life insurance policy was only a good investment as long as you were working there. When you move on to the next job you will have to find new insurance. And then there is the matter of retirement. What happens if once you retire all of your former life insurance policies expire because they were not portable? Yes, "portability" is a very important term used to define a really good life insurance policy. By the same token, a good workplace philosophy is only as good as its portability. Say you worked on a golf course for ten years (like I did years ago in my twenties) and the company's philosophy was "Keep it looking like the green green grass of home." (I just made that up for the sake of argument; wasn't really our motto.) That would be a great philosophy for a golf course; they look the best when they are all green. But how useful is that if your next job or career is at a hospital or university or some type of office building? You see where I'm going with this? It's not much of a portable philosophy. The point is this: Working with God is portable. You can take that philosophy and ministry *anywhere*, even into retirement. This is not to say you should go forth and preach the Gospel to everyone who works with you at the car dealership, the university, or even that new hospital you transferred to. Just take that peace of mind with you wherever you go; better still, the peace of Christ. Allow the Holy Spirit to work in and through you so that co-workers and even strangers can plainly see what a spiritual and righteous (but not self-righteous *please!*) person looks, works and acts like. In this way, and without annoying or disrespecting the people around you, you will truly be working with God. I'd like to end this chapter with a verse from Scripture to send you out into the world of Sterile Processing, much like Jesus sent His disciples into the world to minister. This comes from the Gospel of John, Chapter 14, verses 22-27 (NIV). Jesus was meeting with His disciples one last time the night before His impending death on the cross. He was explaining to them that He was going up to be with His Father and to prepare a place for them in His Father's kingdom. Yet some of them still doubted His words to the very end. Jesus quelled their doubts:

Then Judas (not Judas Iscariot) said, "But, Lord, why do you intend to show yourself to us and not to the world?"

Jesus replied, "Anyone who loves me will obey my teaching. My Father will love them, and we will come to them and make our home with them. Anyone who does not love me will not obey my teaching. These words you hear are not my own; they belong to the Father who sent me."

"All this I have spoken while still with you. But the Advocate, the Holy Spirit, whom the Father will send in my name, will teach you all things and will remind you of everything I have said to you. Peace I leave with you; my peace I give you. I do not give to you as the world gives. Do not let your hearts be troubled and do not be afraid."

May the peace of Christ be with you always.

ABOUT THE AUTHOR

Richard Craig Hughes was born in Willowdale, Ontario, a suburb of Toronto, Canada in the late 1950's. His father Carl (1918-2007) moved the family down to Vero Beach, Florida in the winter of 1966 in the middle of a snowstorm that dropped over 18 inches of snow in their neighborhood in just a few hours. After finally adjusting to the hot Florida climate, as a teenager Richard began picking up hobbies such as surfing, dirt bike racing, and cycling. In the winter of 2008, after graduating from the University of Central Florida with a Bachelor's degree in Psychology, Rick and his wife Kelly moved to Central Florida. He now enjoys playing ice hockey as a goalie at the local ice rink and plans on working as a sterile processing technician until he retires.

www.ingramcontent.com/pod-product-compliance
Lightning Source LLC
Chambersburg PA
CBHW060840170526
45158CB00001B/196